Praise for
From the Heart of a Mother

"We love sharing Randi's poems with our Her View From Home community. Our readers easily relate to her heartfelt words about motherhood. It's the kind of connection we all need. Any mother who reads *From the Heart of a Mother* is sure to find a piece of herself inside."

—**Leslie Means**, bestselling author of *So God Made a Mother* and founder/owner of Her View From Home, LLC

"Reading Randi's poems is like chicken soup to a mother's soul. They're raw, honest, and vulnerable. After reading one, I find myself nodding in agreement or touching my heart like I just had an encouraging and heartfelt conversation with a good friend. I feel seen and comforted. Her words speak to women everywhere, reminding us how beautiful motherhood is while letting us know we aren't alone through the challenging parts. Every mother needs her book."

—**Danielle Sherman-Lazar**, creator of Living Full and author of *It's Okay to Not Be Okay: Adults Get Big Feelings Too*

"Randi's words and poems have been touching my heart for years now. She is able to capture the powerful emotions that come with motherhood and help us feel fully seen, less alone. Randi also shares openly about life's challenges and offers hope and light for the journey. What a gift that her words will now be in a book, able to bless so many more who need them."

—**Sydnei Kaplan**, author of *The Heaven Phone*

"Randi is a true talent, and her words are a balm for a weary mother's soul. They are vulnerable and honest, beautifully capturing this life experience. Without a doubt, Randi will prove to be a literary powerhouse. Many of her quotes are already well-known and beloved across the internet, and I foresee her many readers and followers (not to mention scores of influential writers and content creators) sharing this book far and wide. You hold a smash hit in your hands."

—**Cassie Gottula Shaw**, founder of Girl, I've Got You and author of *Dream Chaser: Live Big, My One Year Old Boy*

"Randi's stunning poetry captures the highs and lows of motherhood with a grace that makes us feel seen. Her words perfectly portray the deep emotions of a mom, particularly how minute-by-minute we can feel blessed and broken and everything in between."

—**Christine Derengowski**, writer

"Randi's encouraging words are what mothers need to get through those long, challenging days and sometimes even longer nights. Her poems are a burst of fresh air, allowing us to feel seen and understood. They touch my heart each and every time."

—**Whitney Fleming**, author and co-owner of Parenting Teens & Tweens

"Randi writes so honestly and openly about the real struggles of life, relationships, and motherhood. She's a truth-teller for women, and that's important. We're all desperate to hear more truth."

—**Mikala Albertson**, MD, author of *Ordinary on Purpose: Surrendering Perfect and Discovering Beauty Amid the Rubble* and *Everything I Wish I Could Tell You About Midlife: A Woman's Guide to Health in the Body You ACTUALLY Have*

"The poetry of Randi Latzman offers a safe landing space for the hearts of all mothers. Her honest, raw, and inspirational words feel universal and yet so personal, as if she's speaking right into the reader's own soul. Her empowering pieces are so needed by mothers today, allowing them to feel their journeys are acknowledged and appreciated. Randi's words are truly a gift."

—**Mehr Lee**, writer at Raise Her Wild

"Randi Latzman is one of my very favorite motherhood writers. She is able to express feelings and experiences that we all walk through and relate to in our journeys raising children. But she does so in such a beautifully poetic way that she leaves her readers nodding their heads in understanding, feeling less alone and validated in their path, and warmed by her artistic expression. Her poems lift and celebrate women in their motherhood as they weave a sense of connection."

—**Emily Roussell**, children's book author of *Rock You Tonight*

"Randi Latzman's words on motherhood will touch every cell in your body. She writes with compassion and grace to remind us all why motherhood is both our greatest and most challenging work."

—**Celeste Yvonne**, author of *It's Not About the Wine: The Loaded Truth Behind Mommy Wine Culture*

"Randi Latzman's poetry not only pays tribute to motherhood, but most importantly, includes every stage and every age. From expectant new moms to the grace of grandmothers, *From the Heart of a Mother* is lyric, lovely, and deeply meaningful. Brava!"

—**Becca Anderson**, bestselling author of *The Book of Awesome Women*

"I am thrilled to wholeheartedly endorse Randi and her incredible writing. Randi has a unique gift for capturing the essence of motherhood, navigating the challenges of parenting, and addressing crucial aspects of mental wellness. Her poetry resonates deeply, offering a genuine and compassionate perspective on the multifaceted journey of motherhood.

"Her ability to tackle topics such as relationships, hardships, and trauma with sensitivity and authenticity sets her apart. Through her words, she provides comfort and understanding for those navigating the complexities of parenthood. Her insights not only shed light on the struggles many face but also offer practical guidance and a sense of solidarity.

"Navigating motherhood is no easy feat, and Randi's poems serve as a beacon of support for mothers everywhere. Whether you're seeking advice, empathy, or simply a moment of reflection, this collection is a must-read.

"In a world where the challenges of parenting can be overwhelming, Randi's writing stands out as a source of inspiration and encouragement. Her poetry is a testament to the strength and beauty found in the shared experiences of motherhood."

—**Jennifer Thompson**, author of *If We're Being Honest*

"Randi's beautiful words help each of us know that we are never alone. She helps us all to see the light in the darkness and the joy in the hard times and the mess. In a world of impossible standards, Randi reminds us we are enough and that we can not only survive but thrive in this season of motherhood, just exactly as we are."

—**Amy Betters-Midtvedt**, educator and author of *You'll Make It and They Will Too: Everything No One Talks About When Parenting Teens*

From the Heart
of a Mother

From the Heart of a Mother

Poetry and Words of Inspiration for All Stages of Motherhood

Randi Latzman

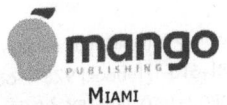

MIAMI

Copyright © 2024 by Randi Latzman.
Published by Mango Publishing, a division of Mango Publishing Group, Inc.

Cover Design: Elina Diaz
Cover Photo/illustration: wacomka/stock.adobe.com
Interior image credit: Nicole Wegman/IG: @art_to_remember_by_nw,
wacomka/stock.adobe.com, GloryStarDesigns/stock.adobe.com
Layout & Design: Elina Diaz

www.survivingmomblog.com

Mango is an active supporter of authors' rights to free speech and artistic expression in their books. The purpose of copyright is to encourage authors to produce exceptional works that enrich our culture and our open society.

Uploading or distributing photos, scans or any content from this book without prior permission is theft of the author's intellectual property. Please honor the author's work as you would your own. Thank you in advance for respecting our author's rights.

For permission requests, please contact the publisher at:
Mango Publishing Group
5966 South Dixie Highway, Suite 300
Miami, FL 33143
info@mango.bz

For special orders, quantity sales, course adoptions and corporate sales, please email the publisher at sales@mango.bz. For trade and wholesale sales, please contact Ingram Publisher Services at customer.service@ingramcontent.com or +1.800.509.4887.

From the Heart of a Mother: Poetry and Words of Inspiration for All Stages of Motherhood

Library of Congress Cataloging-in-Publication number: 2024941634
ISBN: (print) 978-1-68481-610-1, (ebook) 978-1-68481-611-8
BISAC category code: POE023050, POETRY / Subjects & Themes / Family

To my Brielle: You are the reason behind every motherhood poem that I write. Being your mom will always be my life's greatest purpose. Thank you for being my greatest teacher and for motivating me to be the best version of myself each day. If I inspire you even half the amount that you inspire me, I'll know I did something right as your mother. There are no words to express how much I love you, but perhaps this book will give you some insight into my heart. I love you to the moon and back.

To all the mothers (in all forms) who love their child(ren) unconditionally, try their very best, and question if they are good moms: keep loving and keep trying. Your children are lucky to have you, and you are not alone on this wild ride we call motherhood.

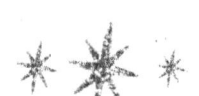

Table of Contents

Foreword	12
From This Mother's Heart	15
Section I—Moms-to-Be and Early Motherhood	19
Section II—Trials and Tribulations of Motherhood	93
Section III—Moms of School-Age and Older Kids	168
Final Musings of My Heart	239
Conclusion	244
Acknowledgements	246
About the Author	250

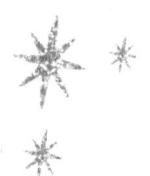

Foreword

I was having a conversation with poet Randi Latzman a few months ago and blurted out, "Well, I'm not a mother, I am only a step-mother," and she reminded me that stepmothers are absolutely parents, too. Rightly so, this engendered some deep thinking for me, reflecting on all the ways I am a mother.

In a marvelous way, Randi prompted me to become more active in my mothering and less passive, which has been wonderful. In fact, the word "*mother*" is both a noun and a verb. It is all those actions, large and small, that create a legacy of love.

Mothers make the world go 'round. People will often ask me if I have a muse or if there is anyone who inspired me to write. Easy answer: my beloved mother, Helen. My mom had to start working immediately upon graduating high school because her dad, my grandfather, passed away and her mother was gravely ill with a rare blood disease. My mom, as a teen, was both a caretaker and breadwinner. If my mother had gotten to attend college—a dream she had to abandon—she would have graduated with every honor as she is brilliant in a very humble and appealing way. Instead, she took care of business and did that brilliantly, too. My mother is an endless inspiration for me;

she encourages me to be kind, work hard, try my best and look out for others, especially women and girls.

The love mothers give to the world extends far beyond the devotion they show their children and families. Moms ensure we have a future through the children they bring into the world so lovingly, to parent, mentor, and guide. Randi Latzman's gorgeous book of poetry, *From the Heart of a Mother*, carries this gift of love in every page and every poem. I will be giving a copy to my mom as one means of thanking her for all she did for me. Thank you, Randi, for creating a fitting tribute to mothers everywhere. Brava!

—**Becca Anderson**, bestselling author

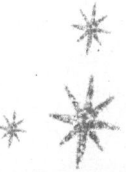

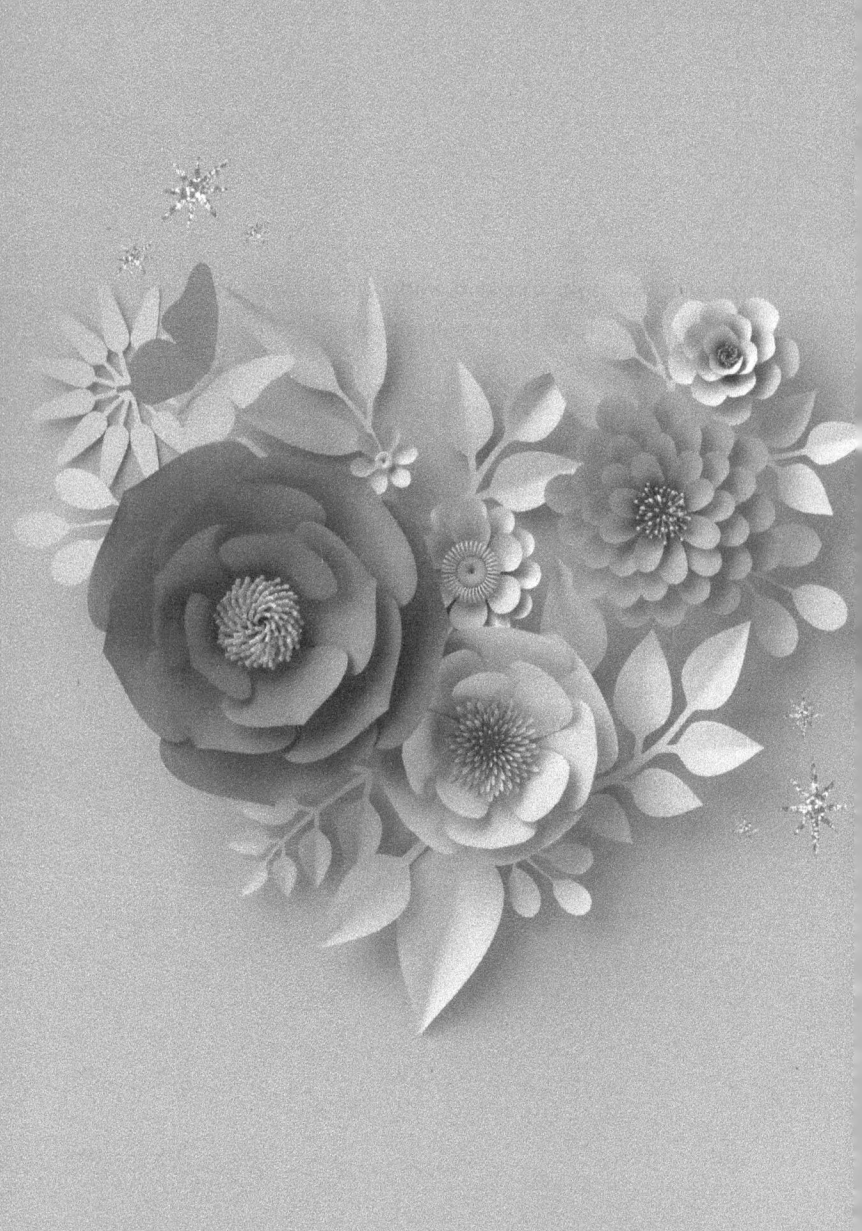

From This Mother's Heart to Yours

Dear Reader,

If you picked up this book, chances are you are a mother or know someone who is. There are various books for moms, so you are probably wondering, "Why should I read this book?" and perhaps also asking, "Are you a parenting expert?"

The answer to that last question is an emphatic "no." I am a mother who often struggles to put one foot in front of the other. I am a mother who second guesses myself and my choices. I am a mother who is far from an expert.

However, I think my answer to the question of whether I am a parenting expert also provides the answer to why you would want to read this book. There are many books out there that claim to have all the answers. I read many of them when I was pregnant. And although I'm not an expert, I speak from experience when I say that you can read all the how-to manuals in the world, but nothing will fully prepare you for the journey of motherhood. There is no one-size-fits-all to parenting.

Mothers often feel alone in their motherhood journey; I know I did. In fact, a Huffington Post survey found that 90 percent of moms are lonely since having children. This percentage illustrates the hard truth that our society does not offer mothers enough emotional support. One of the most frequent comments I get from readers is, "I thought I was the only one who felt that way." There are too many of us silently suffering, not knowing that others are going through the very same struggles we are experiencing. This must stop, and I hope that my book will give moms a much-needed voice and a safe place.

Motherhood has a funny way of showing you all your flaws. Ironically, I also think that is where the beauty of motherhood lies. No matter how often and how hard we try, we are never going to be perfect moms. We are human beings, which means we will make mistakes. However, it is within those imperfections and errors that we discover who we truly are—flawed, complicated, emotional beings with mama hearts that are filled with more love than we ever imagined. Imperfection, effort, and unconditional love are interwoven in my poems, as they are in our lives. My writing comes from this mother's heart to yours, and I hope you find solace in these words.

There are many motherhood poetry books that write about the joys of being a mom, but that approach only touches upon one side of the journey. My child is my greatest blessing and gift, and many of the poems in this book express those sentiments. However, I don't want to just write about how much I love my child (which I do), because motherhood isn't just about love. Motherhood is struggling with loneliness, doubt, uncertainty, worry, and guilt, alongside the positive emotions of love, hope, tenderness, joy, and effort. My poems articulate the highs and lows of motherhood, while describing raw truths, vulnerabilities, and a love that is all-encompassing. It is those complex and often contradictory emotions that are the essence of being a mom, and I explore all of them in this book.

I also want to write about the complete evolution of motherhood, not just the early years. Motherhood is not just until our children are eighteen. We are moms forever, and this book includes all phases of motherhood. Therefore, my book is divided into sections that reflect a cohesive journey. Section I contains poems about revelations and self-discoveries during the early stages of motherhood, while Section II focuses on its trials and tribulations. Section III embarks upon the difficulty and selflessness of letting go of our children as they grow.

My hope is that my book will resonate with you whether you are an expectant mom, stepmom, foster mom, adoptive mom, first-time mom, mom with several kids, mom with one kid, mom of older children, mom of adult children, and/or a grandma. I am writing solely from a mother's perspective, but this book is for you whether you're single, married, separated, widowed, or divorced. I also want to point out that I have a daughter; although the pronouns "she" and "her" are often used, the poems are meant to include any child.

Motherhood often feels like you finally figured it out, only to discover that all the questions changed. It reminds me of a dog chasing its own tail. Children know how to push our buttons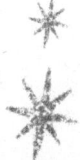

and test us in every way possible. They hold up a mirror to our wounded parts, and they make us question ourselves. You are not alone in feeling that way, and you are not alone in your struggles. If there is one takeaway from my book, it is that a good mom isn't one who does everything right. A good mom is one whose unconditional love and efforts are unwavering.

I often felt like a bad mom because it is easy to look around and feel like everyone else has their life together. Social media often perpetuates that cycle of shame and guilt as we look at picture-perfect families and spotless homes. That sense of shame and guilt isolated me and made me feel like a failure. Motherhood can leave you feeling lonely while you're surrounded by children. I wish there had been a book out there that spoke about the whole motherhood experience, and this is the inspiration behind my writing.

As you read, my sincerest wish is that my poems hold your hand in the valleys of motherhood, cheer you on as you dare the peaks, and support you through all the in-betweens.

From my heart to yours, I hope this book makes you feel seen, heard, and understood.

Love,
Randi

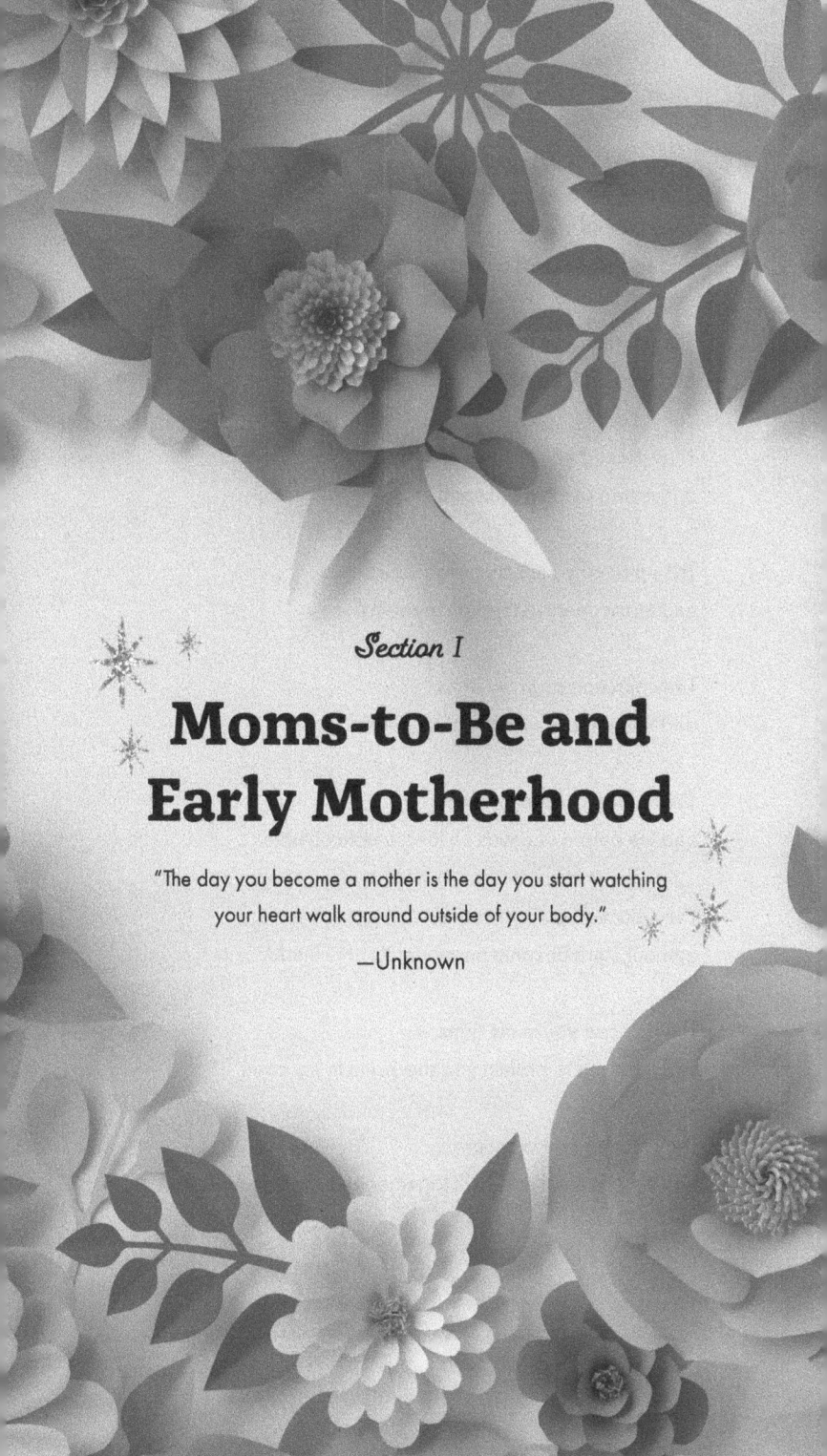

Section I

Moms-to-Be and Early Motherhood

"The day you become a mother is the day you start watching your heart walk around outside of your body."

—Unknown

They Placed You in My Arms

They placed you in my arms,
and suddenly I was a mother.

They placed you in my arms,
and time both slowed down and sped up.

They placed you in my arms,
and a part of me awakened.

They placed you in my arms,
and terror coursed through my veins.

They placed you in my arms,
and the sun rose and set in your eyes.

They placed you in my arms,
and life before you was no longer conceivable.

They placed you in my arms,
and our souls became permanently entwined.

They placed you in my arms,
and the need to protect you shook me to my core.

They placed you in my arms,
and the pieces of my life fit together and shattered all at once.

They placed you in my arms,
and my life had a deeper purpose.

They placed you in my arms,
and I knew everything and nothing.

They placed you in my arms,
and the love I felt was palpable.

They placed you in my arms,
and I was suddenly and forever a mother.

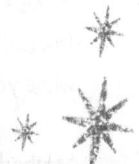

Motherhood Can Feel Lonely

Motherhood can feel lonely.

The cries of your baby
tussle the night's slumber.
The walls of the room
echo the pleading of your heart.

Motherhood can feel lonely.

You cling to memories
of mature interactions.
The only adult voice is within your mind
as you are shackled to your home.

Motherhood can feel lonely.

Your wants and needs
are no longer center stage.
Your dusks and dawns
are collections of giving.

Motherhood can feel lonely.

You feel enormous guilt
for missing life before motherhood.
The isolation is overflowing
while you are submerged by another.

Motherhood can feel lonely.

You try to find a village,
but villages aren't easy to find.
You try to schedule conversations,
but plans are often broken.

Motherhood can feel lonely.

You adore your child
and love being their mother,
but feel pangs of loneliness
and waves of crushing sorrow.

Motherhood can feel lonely.

But there are many mothers
who wrestle with those feelings.
The stirrings of their hearts
beat succinctly with yours.

Motherhood can feel lonely.

If we voice our silent cries,
it can be audible to others.
A light can shine at the end of the tunnel,
if we are willing to share our location.

Motherhood can feel lonely,
but you don't have to do it alone.
Share the melody of your soundtrack
so it can be sung by another.

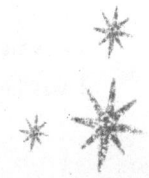

I Was the First

I was the first.

I was the first who held you in my arms
I was the first who wept tears of love
I was the first who rocked you to sleep
I was the first who felt your hand around my finger

I was the first.

I was the first name you spoke
I was the first you walked and ran towards, arms outstretched
I was the first who sang to you
I was the first who whispered words of comfort

I was the first.

I was the first who you came to
when you had something to share
I was the first who you leaned on for reassurance
I was the first who told you stories
I was the first who rubbed your back
and stroked your hair when you felt sick

I was the first.

I was the first who played games with you
I was the first who made you laugh

I was the first who made you feel safe
I was the first whose heart both burst and broke
when you had all your firsts

I was the first.

I was the first who loved you.
I was the first who got to be your whole world.
I was the first who had to let go,
for there are many others who love you
and will be loved by you.

But there will never be anyone who will love you quite like I do
Because I was the first.

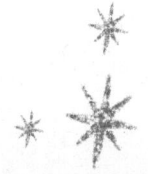

Through It All

I'll wipe away your fallen tears.
I'll offer shelter through your fears.
I pray you know within your soul.
I will love you through it all.

I'll offer an ear to listen.
I'll stand beside you every season.
I'll cheer through the highs,
raise you up when you fall.
Wherever life may take you,
I will love you through it all.

I know the depths of my love
are hard to fully comprehend.
But when you are a parent
you'll finally understand.

You will take your baby's hand,
and feel a love that has no end.
You will see the sun set and rise
each time you look into their eyes.

You'll make mistakes every day.
You'll doubt yourself in every way.
And you'll pray they always know
you will love them through it all.

And I pray you always know
that wherever you may go
I will love you through life's all.
I will love you through it all.

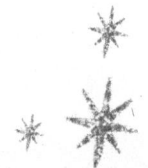

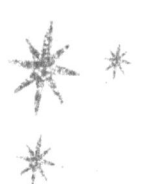

Our Answer

In a world full of uncertainty,
our love for our children
is the one constant we can guarantee

In a world full of questions,
our love for our children
will always be our answer

I Didn't Know Existed

Motherhood showed me parts of myself
that I didn't know existed.

the instinctual need to protect you at any cost
the waves of frustration and guilt
the ultrasonic hearing with every twitch, sound,
and breath you take
the endless second guessing
the way my heart shatters into a million pieces
when you struggle
and how my heart feels like it can burst with love

Motherhood revealed parts of myself that I didn't know existed.

how I yearn to do better and be better for you
how watching you grow causes both grief and intense gratitude
the way I miss you when you're not with me,
while also yearning for moments of solitude
how I feel the constant weight of responsibility to do right by you
the strength I discovered to take care of you,
regardless of my own defeats, illnesses, or hardships
how your joy brings me elation, and your sadness brings me
new depths of sorrow

Motherhood has taught me about parts of myself
that I didn't know existed
and no matter your age, I am forever changed
and forever grateful.

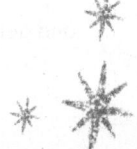

Motherhood Is

Motherhood is tantrums and crying
Motherhood is cuddling and kisses
Motherhood is raised voices and frustration
Motherhood is teachable moments and forgiveness

Motherhood is testing boundaries and pushing buttons
Motherhood is the feel of their hand in yours
Motherhood is endless worry and guilt
Motherhood is big hugs and excited faces

Motherhood is frazzling and exhausting
Motherhood is watching your child's chest rise
and fall in their sleep
Motherhood is unpredictability and uncertainty
Motherhood is finding an inner strength
you didn't know existed

Motherhood is learning to trust your instincts
Motherhood is learning what it means
for your heart to burst with love

Motherhood is the most difficult thing
and the most beautiful thing

Motherhood is giving your child your everything
and getting more than you ever imagined.

You Are Never Alone

I wish I could shield you from all of life's cruelties
but I cannot.

you are going to struggle
you are going to feel pain
you are going to feel heartbreak
you are going to feel sadness
I want you to know that it is normal to experience those feelings

My child,
I cannot protect you
from the harsh realities of this world
but know this...

You are never alone in this world.

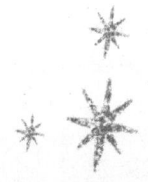

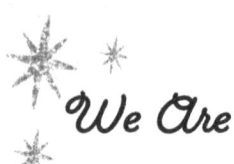
We Are

We are the boo-boo healers
We are the schedule makers
We are the shoulder to lean on
We are the picture takers.

We are the tear driers
We are the warm embrace
We are the whispers of comfort
We are the safe place.

We are the nurturers
We are the number one fans
We are the memory keepers
We are the makers of plans.

We are the hand holders
We are the cheerleaders
We are the voice of reason
We are the life teachers.

We are the guardians
We are the protectors
We are the leaders
We are the earth shakers.

We are the words of truth
We are the hopes for tomorrow
We are the endless possibilities
We are the lifters of sorrow.

We face countless hardships,
but always rise when we fall.
Because a mother's love gives her strength:
the most powerful love of them all.

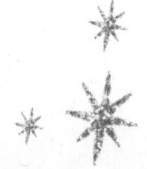

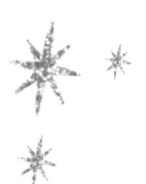

Effort

I want my child to grow up
and know that the hardest things in life
are worth the effort.

Instead of chasing perfection,
I hope she follows her dreams,
loves wholeheartedly,
and always gives it her all.

You Inspire Me

When I first laid eyes on you,
I knew how profoundly my life would change.

And it has.
Because every day,
you inspire me.

you inspire me to be the best version of myself
you inspire me to be open about my emotions
and hold space for them
you inspire me to never give up and to always keep trying

You inspire me.

you inspire me to admit my mistakes and apologize
you inspire me to see beauty within the world
when I am surrounded by darkness
you inspire me to love myself
so that you can unconditionally love yourself

You inspire me.

you inspire me to heal the parts of myself that I've neglected
you inspire me to be more patient and understanding
you inspire me to have courage and strength
when I feel weak and powerless

You inspire me.

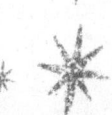

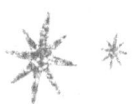

you inspire me to have compassion and empathy
you inspire me to be myself unapologetically
you inspire me to cherish the simple moments in life

You inspire me.

you inspire me to love wholeheartedly and unconditionally
you inspire me to laugh and not take things so seriously
you inspire me to do what is best for my family,
regardless of what others may think

You inspire me.

you inspire me to be a better person and a better mom
you inspire me to grow and evolve
you inspire me to open my heart and love
more than I knew was imaginable

You inspire me in every way.

You inspire me, and you always will.

Firstborn

It was you
whose flutter in my belly
left imprints in my heart.

It was you
whose kick awakened
something deep within my soul.

It was you
who grew within me
as I grew too.

It was you
that felt so unknown,
but also so familiar.

It was you
that showed me
the miracles of my body.

It was you
that left me breathless
as I held you in my arms.

It was you
whose cry from trembling lips
left me in waves of despair.

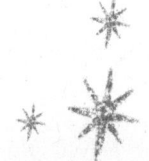

It was you
who showed me
how deeply I could love.

It was you
who first locked eyes with me
and whispered "Mama."

It was you
who gave me
the most humbling and awe-inspiring role.

It was you
who left me with crippling doubt
and endless uncertainty.

It was you that forever changed me.
It was you.
My firstborn.

I'm a Mom

I'm a mom.
Those words sound so simple, but they
carry immeasurable meaning.

I'm helping to shape the life of another human
being in infinite ways, every single day.
I play an integral role in how my child views
and treats herself and others.
I'm her support system, role model, and
source of comfort.

I'm a mom, and I say those words with pride.
For it is the biggest responsibility and honor of my life.

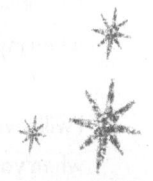

I Will Love You

I will love you
on my darkest days

I will love you
when uncertainty is certain

I will love you
when the worst parts of me awaken

I will love you
when you are in a bottomless hole

I will love you
when I make questionable choices

I will love you
when you push me away

I will love you
irrespective of mistakes made

I will love you
when you reach out for me

I will love you
when my frustrations storm in all directions

I will love you
when you are headstrong and temperamental

I will love you
when the only voice I hear is my own

I will love you
when you lash out with words and choices

I will love you
every second, minute, and hour

with every beat of my heart—
I will love you.

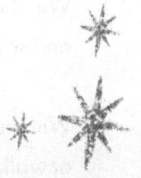

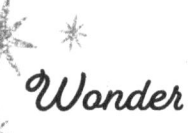

Wonder

I wonder what she'll be like
when she is fully grown.

Will she remember her self-worth
when others try to break her spirit?

Will she grasp the love I have for her,
and that it is unwavering?

Will she lead with the chanting of her heart
rather than the haze of her reflection?

Will she reach for the phone
to hear the tenor of my voice?

Will she follow her inner voice
rather than the path that's simpler?

Will she understand that I made mistakes,
but I always tried my best?

Will she follow her passions and joy,
rather than succumbing to life's pressures?

Will she come to me for advice
and seek my presence?

Will she hold her head up high,
or walk with shoulders slumped?

Will she feel that no matter where she is,
I am always with her in mind and heart?

Will she know that her value
is not based on numbers on a scale?

Will she still see me as her role model
and proudly call me her mom?

Will she share stories with me
and laugh side-by-side?

Will she feel that all roads
will always lead her home?

Will she still seek my warm embrace
and see me as her safe place?

I look at my not-so-little-child,
and I cannot help but wonder.

As the story of her life unwinds,
I wonder if she will ever comprehend
what a wonder she is to me.

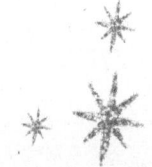

I Will Always Believe in You

From the moment I held you, I worried.
The world can be big and scary,
and my arms wouldn't always be your safe place.
As I rocked you and your eyelashes fluttered,
I prayed you knew.
I will always believe in you.

From the moment you took your first steps,
I held my breath.
Your footprints led to me,
but I knew life would one day take you elsewhere.
Whatever path you forge,
I will always believe in you.

From the moment you cried out in pain,
my heart broke.
I kissed your scrapes,
but my kisses wouldn't heal all of your pain.
Sadness would find its way into your bones,
and I couldn't cast it away.
Whatever heartache you experience,
I will always believe in you.

From the moment you encountered failure,
I felt a pit in my stomach.
There are many challenges you would face,
and your house of cards would eventually collapse.
When disappointment envelops you,
I will always believe in you.

When you feel the ground beneath you tremble,
I pray my love anchors you.
For no matter the choices you make
or the curveballs thrown your way,
I know these words to be true—
I will always believe in you.

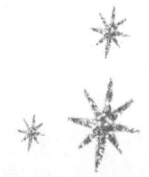

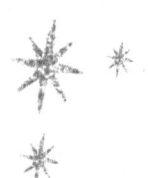

You Are Magic

Even on your worst day,
you are magic
in the eyes of your children.

Your love is everything they need.

How I Love Her Laughter

How I love her laughter.

the laugh that seemed to bounce off every wall
when she was an infant
the laugh that was bigger than her tiny body
the laugh that uplifted me, no matter my mood

How I love her laughter.

the laugh that was often a byproduct of mischief
the laugh that reminded me that what is intangible
is often the most precious
the laugh that could move the highest mountains

How I love her laughter.

the laugh that erupts without reservation
the laugh that accompanies a sparkle in her eyes
the laugh that cannot contain her excitement and joy

And although hardships will inevitably seep into her life,
I pray her laugh will always be around the corner

How I love her laughter.

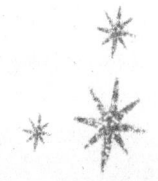

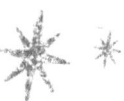

Her laugh is a reminder that there is good in this world
Her laugh is a reminder that I've done something right in this world
Her laugh is the most beautiful sound in this world

Her laugh will always be a balm for my soul

How I love her laughter.

My One and Only

You were my first.
You were my last.
You are my one and only.

It started with you.
It ends with you.
You are my everything.

Each kick.
Each wave of nausea.
Each flutter.

I didn't know then
that every movement
would be my forever.

When I held you in my arms,
my eyes saw color for the first time.
When I heard your cries,
I felt the true meaning of pain.

You sang the name "mama"
and no one else
will chant those lyrics.

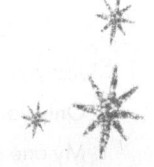

Every milestone was bittersweet,
because that triumph will never
rattle my heart again.

Each chiming of the clock
was the final bell
as the curtain closed.

Guilt tugs at my sleeve
making me wonder
what ifs and why nots.

Grief often floods my heart.
Waves of regret and longing
for what will never be.

Life rolled the dice.
And although I didn't win,
I played the best I could.

I gave you all my heart.
I loved you with all my soul.
For you are my one and only.

I wake for you.
I pray for you.
And I'd die for you.

Just you.
Only you.
My one and only.

Your Worth

Dear Child,

Your worth is like the stars.

It is always there,
even if it cannot be seen.

Your worth is everlasting.

You don't have to do anything
to be worthy.

You already are.
You always were.

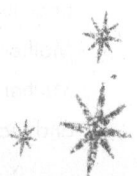

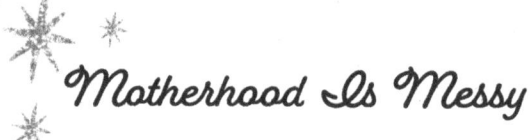
Motherhood Is Messy

Motherhood is messy.

Motherhood is finally locating your kid's shoe
and getting everyone into the car,
only to realize you didn't take your wallet.
Motherhood is trying to convince your child
that they don't need every toy in the store
and the mannequins aren't for touching.
Motherhood is playing the same children's tunes
for the 10,000th time
and resisting the urge to cover your ears.

Motherhood is messy.

Motherhood is yearning to use the bathroom
without an audience.
Motherhood is your child getting into your makeup
and dropping eyeshadow all over the bathroom floor.
Motherhood is pandemonium, exhaustion,
and endless amounts of cleaning.

Motherhood is messy.

Motherhood is eye-rolling, door slamming,
and muttering under their breaths.
Motherhood is testing your patience and possibly your sanity.
Motherhood is feeling endless guilt
and second guessing your decisions.

Motherhood is messy.

Motherhood is worrying about your kids, no matter their age.
Motherhood is challenging, frustrating, and full of hurdles.
Motherhood is putting one foot in front of the other
and falling several times along the way.

Motherhood is messy
and filled with laughter, tenderness, and unconditional love.
Motherhood is bracing yourself for the bumps
and savoring the peaks.
Motherhood is trying to embrace the chaos
and cherishing the moments that bring unimaginable joy.

Motherhood is messy, but the love...
Oh, that love.

Motherhood is a beautiful mess,
and it is the greatest ride of my life.

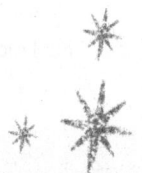

I Didn't Realize

I knew being a parent was hard
but I didn't realize it was the hardest thing I'd ever do

I knew that I would worry
but I didn't realize how much my heart would ache

I knew I would make mistakes
but I didn't realize how often I would make them

I knew that I would be exhausted
but I didn't realize physical weariness would turn emotional

I knew I had a lot to learn about motherhood
but I didn't realize nothing could prepare me for it

I knew that you would need me
but I didn't realize how much I'd need you

I knew that I'd question my choices
but I didn't realize that guilt would be my shadow

I knew that I would love you
but I didn't realize that love would be so powerful

I knew that there would be challenges
but I didn't realize that each age has its own roadblocks

I knew that I would teach you
but I didn't realize that you would be my greatest teacher

I knew that my life would change
but I didn't realize that you would forever change me.

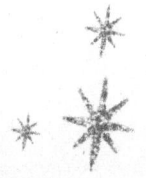

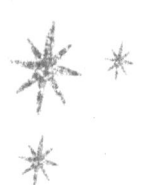

Tomorrow

Hug your kids
a little tighter

Play with them
a little longer

Tell the people you love
how much they mean to you

Because we never know
what tomorrow may bring

Always Be

You'll always be my reason why
You'll always be my source of pride
I'll always be there heart and soul
I'll always be your hand to hold

I am always a part of you
You are always a part of me
We will always be connected
from now to eternity.

You'll always be my greatest strength
You'll always be the breath I take
I'll always be your biggest fan
I'll always be your place to land

I am always a part of you
You are always a part of me
We will always be connected
from now to eternity.

You'll always be my source of worry
You'll always be my favorite story
I'll always question and second guess
I'll always feel so very blessed

I am always a part of you
You are always a part of me
We will always be connected
from now to eternity.

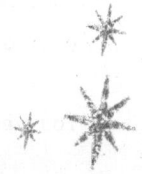

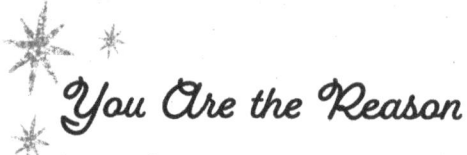

You Are the Reason

You are the reason.

you are the reason my heart feels like it will burst with love
you are the reason I get out of bed each morning,
no matter my exhaustion
you are the reason I feel blessed beyond measure and words

You are the reason.

you are the reason I strive to be the best version of myself
you are the reason I question my choices
you are the reason I never go to bed without feeling guilty

You are the reason.

you are the reason I put one foot in front of the other
you are the reason I know
the true meaning of unconditional love
you are the reason I keep showing up

You are the reason.

you are the reason I both celebrate
and grieve memories passed
you are the reason I admit my mistakes
you are the reason I feel everything you feel a thousandfold

You are the reason.

you are the reason I worry endlessly
you are the reason I will never stop trying
you are the reason I am inextricably changed

You are my reason,
and I am so grateful to be your mom—
always.

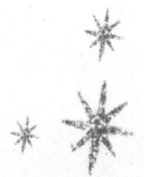

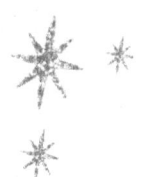

Love Unlike Any Other

It is love unlike any other

It is unaffected by age,
location,
or life circumstances

It is all-consuming
It is everlasting
It is unconditional

Words cannot do it justice,
for it leaves a permanent imprint
on your heart

It is a mother's love.

With You

I may not always say the right thing,
but I always love you
I may not always do the right thing,
but I always love you

In a world where life is uncertain,
the one certainty is my love for you

No matter what you say
No matter what you do
My love will always be with you

Always.

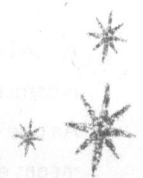

Numbers

Numbers are a concept
we teach to our kids when they are small.
But numbers take up increasing space
in our hearts and minds.

Numbers are used to determine
first height, weight, and time of birth.
Numbers are used to record
dates of milestones and firsts.

Numbers are used to measure
the dimensions of an object.
Numbers are used to count
and for phone numbers and address.

Along the way these numbers
hold different meaning and value.
Along the way these numbers
are used to reflect a person's meaning and value.

An IQ of 90
means below average intelligence.
The numbers on tests
determine our mastery of a subject.

A number on a report card
is associated with pride or shame.
An age above a certain number
means elderly and frail.

A number above a certain weight
is often paired with judgment.
A number below a certain weight
is often paired with judgment.

In a world filled with numbers,
we forget what matters most.
In a world filled with numbers,
we focus on the wrong things.

A number on a scale
won't measure my kindness.
The number on my pants
doesn't reflect if I exercise.

A number on a quiz
doesn't mirror intelligence.
The age one masters tying shoes
doesn't indicate a love of walking.

A 90-year-old might be filled with life,
while a 20-year-old can be filled with pain.
My child took an extra six months to potty train,
but does it really matter?

Numbers are just one measurement.
Just one determination of acuity.
They are a guideline,
but they don't have to be our lifeline.

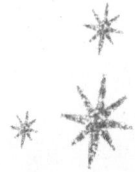

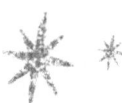

For there is so much in this life
that we cannot measure.
There is so much in this world
that cannot be constrained by a number.

Numbers do not define us.
Numbers don't measure our worth.

We all are filled with light,
and that which makes us shine cannot be quantified.

I Have No Idea What I Am Doing

I have no idea what I am doing.

Those thoughts raced through me like adrenaline.
I held my newborn baby who wouldn't stop crying,
and I felt an overwhelming sense of defeat.

This tiny, helpless baby
was counting on me to take care of her.
This little glimpse of heaven
was counting on me for answers.

And I had none.
For I had no idea what I was doing.

I was told that cries meant different things,
but all her cries belted out the same melody.
I would feed her, burp her, and change her,
only to have her start crying again.

Did she need more food?
Was my supply enough?
Is she getting enough sleep?
Is she getting too much sleep?

I was told her weight was great
and that I was doing everything correctly.

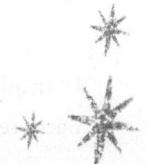

But that couldn't be true.
Because I had no idea what I was doing.

She would stay up during the night
when I was so tired I could barely move.
She would sleep through everything during the day
when I was so tired I couldn't sleep.

She smelled like innocence,
and her skin was as soft as silk.
The love I felt for her was palpable,
but I was terrified of failing her.

Because I had no idea what I was doing.

Days turned into weeks that turned into months.
She eventually slept throughout the night.
And although we settled into a routine,
I still felt the weight of the world on my shoulders.

Because I had no idea what I was doing.

At the same time I also wanted to hit rewind
and freeze frames,
where the whispers of words
and whooshes of the rocking chair
reverberated alongside the beating of her heart.

I craved her presence, but fear still rattled my veins.
Because I had no idea what I was doing.

I watched her many firsts
and was mesmerized by them all.
And when she smiled at me
the birds sang louder and the sun shone brighter
for the world smiled with her.

Still, I had no idea what I was doing.

But then she looked at me,
arms stretched and said, "Mama."
That simple word stopped me in my tracks.
Because of all the words she could say,
and all the people she could choose,
my baby chose my name
to speak through parted lips.

I had no idea what I was doing.
Perhaps I never would.

But when she was born,
my love traveled through my chest and into hers,
where it would forever make a home.

That was enough.
And that was everything.

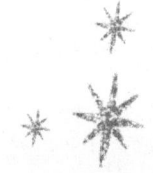

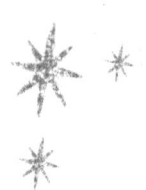

Greatest Power

Dear Moms,

Our greatest source of power
isn't our looks,
our smarts,
our popularity,
or our wealth

The greatest power each of us has
is found within our hearts

What a wonderful world it would be
if we all tapped into that power

I Met a Girl

I met a girl,
and a veil was lifted from my eyes.
Spectrums of hues danced upon a blackened pane.

I met a girl,
and she chased away my demons.
My pain was channeled into purpose.

I met a girl,
and she mended my soul.
Love now pounded through my heart.

I met a girl,
and she gave me strength.
Hardships were no match for her smile.

I met a girl,
and I questioned everything.
Her safety and stability were my only truth.

I met a girl,
and my priorities shifted.
Each day began and ended with her.

I met a girl,
and I knew the meaning of fear.
The thought of failing her brought me to my knees.

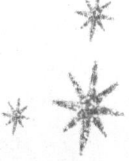

I met a girl,
and she gave me life
the moment I became her mother.

The Worth of a Mother

The worth of a mother cannot be measured by income,
because there isn't a salary.
The worth of a mother cannot be measured by bonuses,
for there are none to receive.
We are not afforded sick, vacation, or mental health days,
although we assuredly need them.

It often feels like the worth of a mother is unquantifiable,
because there is no way of measuring it.
It often feels like a mother's efforts are overlooked,
because there are no performance reviews.
It often feels like a mother's tasks are trivialized,
because there is no promotion or prior experience required.

The makings of a mother cannot be itemized,
but not because the list is too small.
Rather, it is because she pours her heart and soul
into her children every single day.
And although we'd love a "thank you" or a "great job"
for all we do,
we continue to mother and shower our children with love,
no matter the lack of accolades.

We cannot measure a mother's worth,
because there are no numbers big enough
to fully encapsulate it.
We cannot give a mother a promotion,
because she has already climbed insurmountable heights
the moment she looks into her child's eyes
and that love spreads into every cell of her body.

We may not get sick days or receive awards,
but we get something with which no other job can compete.
We are paid in love.
And that love is priceless.

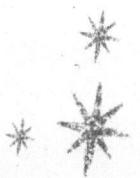

Some Days

Some days I'm a frazzled mom
filled with a sense of unease.
Some days I'm a tired mom
counting down till I get my ZZZs.

Some days I'm a flexible mom.
I'm able to go with the flow.
Some days I'm a funny mom
better than a comedy show.

Some days I'm a serious mom
unable to join in the fun.
Some days I'm a sluggish mom.
Simple tasks are left undone.

Some days I'm a creative mom
art projects and crafts galore.
Some days I'm an organized mom
cleaning from ceiling to floor.

I'm not just one kind of mom
because life changes constantly.
But my love, a mother's love—
that's the one thing I can guarantee.

Time

The greatest gift
we can give our children
is our time

It doesn't cost us a thing,
but its value is priceless

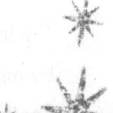

From the Heart of a Mother

The saying is one wears their heart on their sleeve,
but that does not capture a mother's heart.
For when a mother breathes life into her child,
her heart has life blown into it as well.

A heart reshaped to fit the depths
of love contained within it.
A heart so filled with breaks and bursts
it appears to expand in size.

And with each first and last
a mother's heart will sink and swell.
And with each moment in-between
a mother's heart will skip a beat.

The heart of a "good" mother
is defined by its unconditional love.
A love that's pure and endless.
The rarest cut of stones.

A heart with bumps and bruises
from all it has endured.
A heart that sparkles and glows
from all the light it casts.

The heart of a mother cannot be judged
by mistakes or imperfections.
For the journey of motherhood
is filled with bumps and roadblocks.

The strength of a mother's heart
is how it stands apart.
The willingness to rise and stand
no matter the rage of the storm.

Endless paths and roads
will birth a mother's heart.
Endless choices and uncertainties
from which it beats and pumps.

No matter the age or situation
a mother's heart pulses to that of her child.
Because it is from the heart of a mother
that we discover the greatest truth—

A mother's heart is unlike any other.

The most beautiful heart is that of a mother.

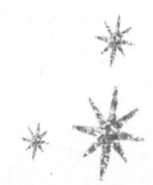

I Feel Everything, My Child

I feel everything, my child.

I feel love as I watch your chest rise and fall in your sleep
I feel guilty for the mistakes that I've made
I feel elation as you laugh and smile

I feel everything.

I feel exasperated when you won't listen
I feel awed when I watch you face your fears
I feel sad that I can't turn back time with you

I feel everything.

I feel worried about whether I'm doing right by you
I feel proud when you try your best
I feel annoyed at myself for losing my temper

I feel everything.

I feel exhausted from the demands of motherhood
I feel honored when your eyes scan for mine across a room
I feel heartache when you are struggling

I feel everything.

I feel the highest highs and the lowest lows
throughout motherhood
Because being a mother has tested me in every way possible
Because I love you more than I ever dreamed was imaginable

I feel everything, my child,
and I always will.

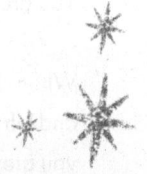

You

In the stillness of the night,
I always think of you.

How your smile breathes life into my soul.
How your laughter radiates brighter than the sun.
How your tears cast daggers into my heart.

When whispers of memories
dance across my mind,
the shadows of those images
will always be of you.

Pangs of guilt
for sharp words that escaped my mouth.
A force that lifts me up
and brings me to my knees.
A love that splatters my heart
and sears it together again.

When I have more questions than answers,
my unspoken prayers will always be you.

For you are the strength that gets me out of bed.
You are the medicine for every ailment.
You are the light at the end of every tunnel.

When down is up
and left is right,
you are my gravity.

You are the promise to every uncertainty.
You are the love that has no ending.
You are the voice when all is silent.

You are the beginning to all my endings.
You are the destination to every journey.

You are my everything, my child.
You.

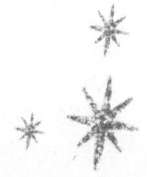

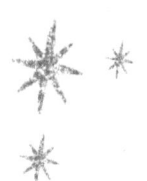

What Is Motherhood?

Motherhood is
loving
with all of your heart,
trying
with all of your might,
and praying
each day
that you're doing it right.

Lastborn

Your lastborn closes the book to your favorite story.
A part of you doesn't want it to be over,
but you know that it is time.

You savor everything more,
because you'll never experience it again.
You feel sadness more,
because you'll never experience it again.
And you feel a new type of guilt,
because you can't give all of yourself to them.

You already know the tricks,
but chances are they don't work with this child.
You already know the answers,
but there is a new set of questions.

You realize your heart has the capacity
to expand with love.
You realize your guilt has the capacity
to multiply and continue.

The clock seems to slow down
and quicken at the same time.
For every first is a last,
and every last is a last.

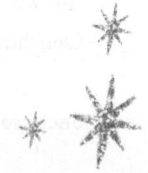

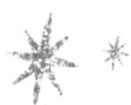

The track plays the same chorus,
although the rhythm varies.
You want to hum along,
while trying to memorize each note.

The clock ticks by, reminding you
that nothing is forever.
The years go by, reminding you
that their childhood isn't forever.

You feel complete,
yet torn apart as well.
Every ounce of sweetness
stings your tongue.

You hope and pray
that you loved them well enough.
You hope and pray
that you were good enough.

The final countdown began
the moment you held them in your arms.
But you loved them just as fiercely.
And you cared just as deeply.

This was a special love story.
One that ended before it even began.

Because this was your lastborn.

Every Day

Every day she grows one day older
Every day I marvel at the child before me

Every day I stumble and feel like I'm failing
Every day I feel blessed to be her mom

Every day she challenges me and pushes my buttons
Every day she inspires me to be better

Every day I question my choices
Every day I try my hardest

Every day I feel waves of frustration
Every day I hope she knows how deeply she is loved

Every day I wonder if I've done enough
Every day she brings a smile to my face

Every day I try to harness her strong will
Every day I am amazed by her wit and determination

Every day I hope parenting gets easier
Every day I wish I could turn back the hands of time

Every day I am filled with guilt and worry
Every day I am filled with love and gratitude

Every day I am reminded of who she once was
Every day I get glimpses of who she is becoming

Every day my heart both grows and shatters
as I navigate the beauty and difficulties of motherhood.

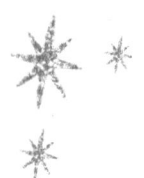

Parenthood

Parenthood is a balancing act
of trying to catch our children
when they fall
while giving them the space to stumble and
find their own footing

The Most Precious Gift

The most precious gift I can give to my child
isn't worth any money

It is something that cannot be touched,
but it is something I pray she always feels

It is with her no matter her age,
no matter her location,
no matter the circumstance

It is unwavering,
everlasting,
and unconditional

It is my love

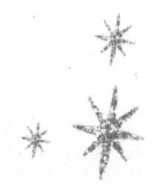

My Greatest Privilege

what a privilege it is to wrap you in my arms
what a privilege it is to be the one you turn to for guidance
what a privilege it is to be your biggest fan

what a privilege it is to hold your hand
what a privilege it is to be your source of comfort
what a privilege it is to be the one you search for
across a crowded room

what a privilege it is to assuage your fears
what a privilege it is to be the one who gives you advice
what a privilege it is to be your role model

what a privilege it is to watch you grow
what a privilege it is to make you feel safe
what a privilege it is to have a front row seat
as you discover yourself

And when the day comes when you spread your wings and fly,
I hope you know that being your mom
will always be my greatest privilege.

There Wasn't Enough Time

Goodbye to tiny fingers that reached out for mine.
Goodbye to wispy hairs that tickled my face.
Goodbye to mobiles and swooshing of rocking chairs.

There wasn't enough time.

Goodbye to bouncers and light up toys.
Goodbye to walkers and night lights.
Goodbye to cries that faded with my kiss.

There wasn't enough time.

Goodbye to fairy tales and stories of wonder.
Goodbye to dolls and dress up clothes.
Goodbye to tiny feet that dangle from chairs.

There wasn't enough time.

Goodbye to endless chatter and squeals of delight.
Goodbye to hide and seek and hopscotch.
Goodbye to coloring books and scribbles on paper.

There wasn't enough time.

Goodbye to play dough and paint by number.
Goodbye to tricycles and training wheels.
Goodbye to nursery rhymes and lullabies.

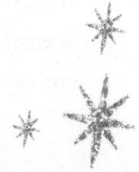

There wasn't enough time.

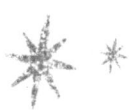

Goodbye to being your sun, moon, and stars.
Goodbye to aches that were only physical.
Goodbye to car seats and child menus.

There wasn't enough time.

Tears fall for what has passed.
An ache for what only exists in my heart.
Memories that feel like yesterday and long ago.

There wasn't enough time.

The struggles that accompanied each day
are saturated by the sharpness of those years.
A perception only visible in the rearview mirror.

The brightest feathers remain from an empty nest.
Time that seemed so slow now seems so very fast.
Walls filled with thunder now deafened by silence.

There wasn't enough time.

There never will be enough time
to savor each version of you.

There never will be enough time
to embrace each wave
and grieve the fall of the tides.

I Would Tell Myself

If I could go back
to the early stages of motherhood
and talk to myself,
there is much I would say.

I would tell myself
that I was doing great,
because fear whispered my name all the time

I would tell myself
that it is impossible to have all the answers
because parenting is an endless journey without any directions

I would tell myself
that the sleepless nights will end,
although it seemed like exhaustion was my constant companion

I would tell myself
that it is okay to miss the days before motherhood,
because it was simpler and less heart-wrenching

I would tell myself
that the days would seem to last forever,
but the years would feel like minutes

I would tell myself
that each stage doesn't get easier.
It is simply a different set of challenges

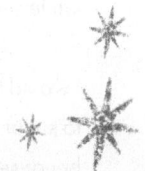

I would tell myself
not to feel pressure to enjoy it all,
because motherhood is filled with highs and lows

I would tell myself
to hold my baby for as long as I want,
because there is no way to gauge the ending of that chapter

I would tell myself
to trust my own instincts,
because nobody knows my child like I do

I would tell myself
that sleepless nights of songs and swaying
were the merging of the hardest and most precious times

I would tell myself
that milestones are just a guideline,
and her laughter and joy are more important

I would tell myself
to be in more photos regardless of appearance,
because those images will leave an imprint on my heart

I would tell myself
that my child will bring out the best in me
while shining a mirror on the worst in me

I would tell myself
to savor the simple moments with her,
because those are the most memorable of them all

I would tell myself
that my unconditional love and efforts
are what matter most

I would tell myself
that I will constantly grieve who my child was
while opening my arms for who she is becoming

I would tell myself
that I am far stronger and more capable
than I ever realized

I would tell myself
that being a mom
would test me in ways I never imagined

I would tell myself
that nothing lasts forever
except for the love between parent and child

I would tell myself
that mistakes are par for the course,
and perfection merely sets me up for failure

I would tell myself
to be kinder to myself
because my child sees more than I realize

I would tell myself
that people will always question my choices
and that shouldn't stop me from making them

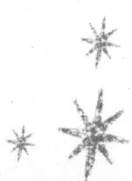

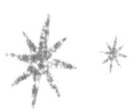

I would tell myself
that motherhood is isolating,
and I will feel my loneliest during those early years

I would tell myself
that the exhaustion transforms
from physical to mental

I would tell myself
that my child will face challenges,
but I will be her greatest advocate

I would tell myself
that I already knew all I needed to know
even though I felt like I knew absolutely nothing

I would tell myself
that I'm raising a remarkable child,
and every difficult moment will be worth it.

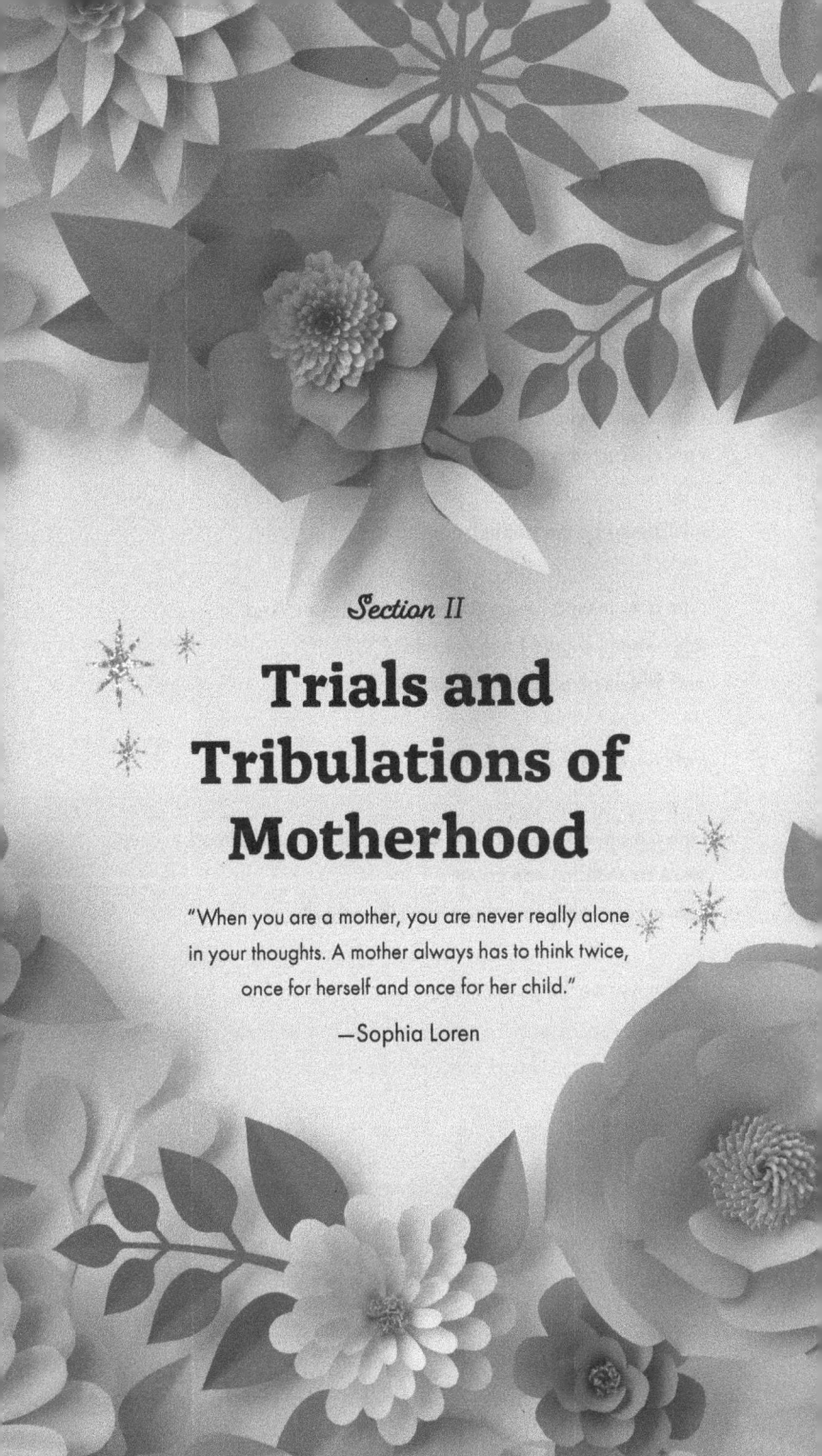

Section II

Trials and Tribulations of Motherhood

"When you are a mother, you are never really alone in your thoughts. A mother always has to think twice, once for herself and once for her child."

—Sophia Loren

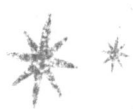

I Will Never Be the Perfect Mom

I will never be the perfect mom.

I am a mom who gets frustrated when I should be more patient
I am a mom who makes mistakes and then makes them again
I am a mom who messes up all the time

I will never be the perfect mom.

I am a mom who listens when I should have talked,
talks when I should have listened,
and makes an already bad situation worse

I will never be the perfect mom.

I am a mom who is frazzled, anxious, and overwhelmed
more times than I can count
I am a mom who doesn't have all the answers

I will never be the perfect mom.

I am an imperfect mom that will always go to bed praying
I did right by my child
I am an imperfect mom that will always show up
I am an imperfect mom that always wears my heart on my sleeve
I am an imperfect mom that loves my child with all my heart
I am an imperfect mom who is full of flaws
but will always keep trying

I will never be the perfect mom.

And I wouldn't change a thing.

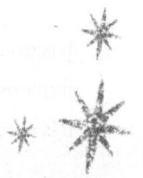

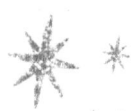

The Mental Load of Motherhood

There is an invisible aspect of motherhood
that often gets ignored.
Although it cannot be seen,
it firmly plants its roots in a mother's brain.

It is the mental load
that is often coupled
with the role of being a mother.

It is knowing, planning, and recalling
every aspect of our child's life.
It is juggling, organizing, preparing,
anticipating, reminding, and formulating.
It is being the CEO, secretary, CFO,
and event planner all in one.

There is a constant barrage of thoughts
racing through our mind at once.
And if you pause or shut it off
for even a moment
you risk expunging
everything you must remember.

It is an alarm
that never shuts off.
It is a constant voice

that only you can hear.
It is an exhaustion
surpassing anything physical.
For it resides in the very recesses of your mind.

You may have a great partner
who takes on chores and duties with you.
But often only one carries that mental load.
And it usually falls upon mothers.

The mental load of motherhood is an invisible weight.
And it's okay if you want someone else to pick it up.
Because it is truly one of the hardest parts of motherhood.

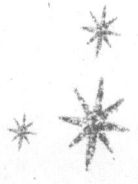

When Life Gets Rough

When life gets rough,
I remind myself that
I brought a beautiful soul
into this world

Every time I look
into her eyes,
I am filled with pride

Every time she
takes my hand,
I am filled with joy

I have a child whom I love
with all my heart

I have everything.

We Are Mothers

There are days when I feel like I can't catch my breath.
There are days when I struggle to get out of bed.
There are days when all I want to do is run and hide.

But I don't fall down that rabbit hole
because I have little eyes and little hands waiting for me.

I have someone who depends on me.
I have someone who looks to me for guidance.
I have someone who seeks me for comfort.

That doesn't mean that I suppress my feelings.
That doesn't mean my emotions disappear.
But it gives me the conviction and determination to get through it.

I struggle.
Yet I keep putting one foot in front of the other,
no matter what life throws my way.
I navigate life's hardships
while guiding my child through her own.

Because motherhood shows us who we really are.
It allows us to discover an inner strength
that we didn't know existed.

We are brave.
We are strong.
We are capable.
We are survivors.

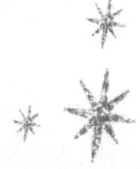

We are mothers.

What Could Have Been

A seed was planted in her mind
that never grew in form.
A light flickered in her heart,
but never quite caught fire.

She gently rubs her belly.
A womb of promise—
now a vessel for pain.
A hollow shell of silence
whispering sounds she'll never hear.

A door slammed in her face
that once was wide and welcome.
Dreams she dared to dream
now cries of shattered heartache.

Grief clutches at her throat
for a reach exceeding her grasp.
Waves of sorrow for what could have been.
Waves of anger for what was taken away.

She carved a path along the gravel,
but the wind blew it away.
A lifetime in her mind
was stolen with a moment's breath.

A question without answers.
A step that was never taken.
The world might have shifted
if what could have been existed.

In the still of the night
she etches her fingers across her belly.
For the one that spoke in her heart,
but never made a sound.

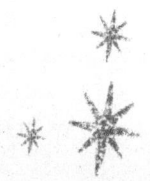

Good Moms

Good moms feel guilty
Good moms try their best
Good moms make mistakes

Good moms struggle
Good moms yearn for moments of solitude
Good moms get frustrated

Good moms may not mother the way you do
Good moms get frazzled
Good moms don't have all the answers

Good moms worry
Good moms love their kids unconditionally
Good moms have flaws

In case you need reminding, you are a good mom.

Am I Doing This All Wrong?

"Am I doing this all wrong?"

My daughter runs upstairs,
the slam of the door echoing throughout the house

"Am I doing this all wrong?"

Explaining to her yet again
that she can't leave her stuff all over the floor

"Am I doing this all wrong?"

Overwhelmed by the emotional, physical,
and psychological needs
of another human being

"Am I doing this all wrong?"

With every wave of frustration, exhaustion, guilt,
uncertainty, and anger

"Am I doing this all wrong?"

A knowing smile on your face when I tell you that I love you.
A rolling of your eyes when I smother you in kisses.
A look of contentment as you drift off to sleep.
A leaning on my shoulder as you sit next to me.

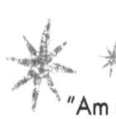 "Am I doing this all wrong?"

You know how deeply you are loved.
Despite all my shortcomings,
what truly matters is being done right.

This Is for the Women

This is for the women who are not mothering like their moms
the ones that didn't get unconditional love growing up
the ones that are forging their own paths

This is for the women who are cycle breakers
who are healing wounds from their childhood
who are trying to be the mothers they never had

This is for the women who didn't have good role models
who must figure motherhood out for themselves
who look at mothers with their own mothers,
and their hearts break

This is for the women that don't have any support
who don't have grandparents that will be there in a pinch
who have constant reminders of what was lacking
in their own upbringing

Your self-awareness makes you a good mom
Your desire to do things differently makes you a good mom
Your willingness to fight your trauma head-on
makes you a good mom

You are giving your children the life and love you never had
You are giving your children the life and love
you deserved to have

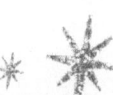

For all those women,
always remember—
you are a good mom.

You are a force to be reckoned with
because it stopped with you.

We Feel

Every scrape that our children feel,
we feel

Every tear that our children cry,
we feel

Every heartache that our children feel,
we feel

Every illness that our children have,
we feel

When you're a mother,
you feel your children's pain exponentially

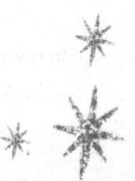

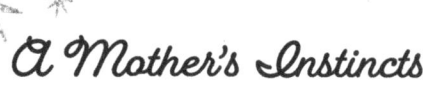
A Mother's Instincts

There are many ways to raise a child.

And there are many people
who want to tell you how you should raise your child.

Some will offer their opinions when asked,
but many will give unsolicited advice.

It is easy to doubt your parenting decisions
when you are surrounded by people questioning your choices.

The truth is what works for one child
may not work for another child.

The truth is what works for one mother
may not work for another mother.

The truth is that every day with your child
is the first day of raising your child at that age.

The truth is that nobody has all the answers.

In a world full of voices,
a mother must trust her instincts.

In a world full of opinions,
a mother must trust her own voice and heart.

A mother may not always get it right,
but a good mother will always do her best.

Stand by your choices
even if others don't agree.

Because a mother's heart
is forever connected to her child.

Trust your intuition,
because you are the parent.

Everyone else is simply white noise.

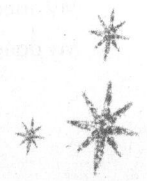

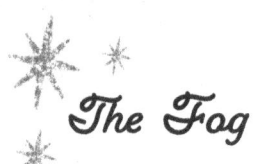

The Fog

After I kissed my daughter goodnight, I sat on the couch to think.
I reflected upon the things I wish I could undo.
The opportunities I had to be more patient.
The times I rushed to judgment instead of rushing to understand.

The ways I could have been a better mom.

As my thoughts continued to wander, the guilt engulfed me.
I felt as though I was in a fog, unable to see.
As the waves of regret washed over me, I closed my eyes.
I took a deep breath and searched deep within my heart.

I heard my daughter's belly laugh when I told her a joke.
I recalled how she snuggled closer to me
as I read her a bedtime story.
I felt her hand finding its way into mine as we walked together.
I imagined her squeal of delight as we played a game.
I saw the look on her face when I kissed her forehead.

And as quickly as it came, the fog cleared.
I was finally able to see what was right in front of me.

I will never do everything correctly, and that's okay.

My daughter doesn't need a perfect mom.
My daughter needs me.

We All Get Lost

As moms, we all get lost sometimes.

Keep caring
Keep trying
Keep going

When our north star is an open mind
and an open heart,
we will always find our way back home.

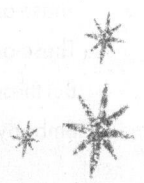

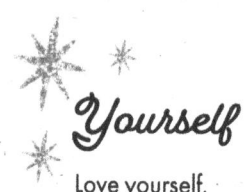

Yourself

Love yourself.

particularly on the days when
you can barely muster the strength
to peel yourself out of bed

Believe in yourself.

even when the world says you can't
especially when you feel like
you're both fading away and sinking

Care for yourself.

when there's barely time to breathe
when every second you are being pulled
in endless directions

Befriend yourself.

when you've fought with others
when you've battled yourself
when you feel like you're alone in a room full of faces

These are easy words to say.
These are easy words to write.
But these little words
embody lifelong inner struggles.

Being a mother is hard enough.
Please.
Remember to be kind to yourself.

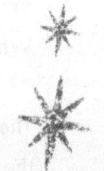

The Worry of a Mother

The worry of a mother
is all-consuming and never-ending.

It gnaws at her mind
the moment her child is placed in her arms.

An endless concern
about every facet of her child.

Is she getting enough to eat?
Is he getting enough sleep?

Did I burp her enough?
What does his cry mean?

Why isn't she walking yet?
Why isn't he talking yet?

Why did I lose my patience again?
Why did I raise my voice again?

Does he know how much I love him?
Does she know how much I love her?

Why isn't she home yet?
Why hasn't he called yet?

They plague her regardless of
the time, location, or age of her child.

For the well-being and safety of her child
are always her utmost priorities.

And whether her child is a baby,
or has kids of their own,
a mother will worry about her child.

Because the worry of a mother
is tethered to her heart.

And her heart
is always with her children.

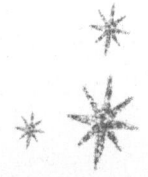

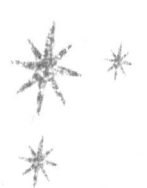

Choice of Motherhood

Motherhood is a choice each and every day
to get yourself out of bed
no matter your own struggles or hardships
to be a role model and teacher
through whatever life throws at them and you
to soar through the highs
and brace yourself through the lows
to love without fear or reservation,
and to give them everything you've got

The Answer Is Love

Mothers are often our own worst critics.
We look at ourselves and immediately notice all the flaws.
We beat ourselves up for what we say and what we do.
We tell ourselves that we aren't good enough mothers, wives,
sisters, daughters, friends...

Why do we tell our children to be kinder to themselves
when we are so cruel to ourselves?
We would never speak to other people
the way we speak to ourselves.
But somehow, the most vile, hurtful words sift through our brains.

We are our own worst enemy.
Focusing on our mistakes.
Feeling endless cycles of shame and guilt.
Kicking ourselves again and again.

Why is it so hard to see the best parts of ourselves?
Why is our inner voice our worst critic?
Why is it so easy to feel self-contempt rather than self-love?

It must stop.
We must stop.

Stop self-judging.
Stop self-loathing.
Stop self-criticizing.
Stop comparing.

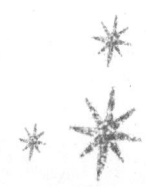

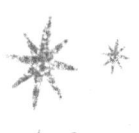

Stop.
Stop.

We must stop.
Hate begets hate.

The answer will always be love.

Love our children.
Love one another.
Love ourselves.

Love.
Love.

It is time to choose love.

The answer will always be love.

Mothers Show Up

Mothers show up.
We show up to recitals
We show up to sporting events
We show up to school plays

Mothers show up.
We show up when we're tired
We show up when we're overwhelmed
We show up when we are filled
with uncertainty and self-doubt

Mothers show up.
We show up with support
We show up with encouragement
We show up with pride

Mothers show up.
We show up when we apologize for our wrongdoings
We show up when we strive to do better for our children
We show up when we juggle schedules, appointments,
and to-do lists

Mothers show up.
And we'll make countless mistakes
We'll stumble and we'll crash
We'll question ourselves along the way

But mothers show up
because no matter our faults or life circumstances
we always show up—
with unwavering love.

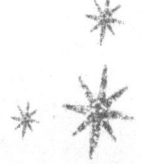

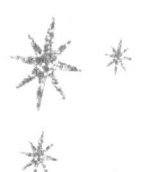

Biggest Paradox of Motherhood

The biggest paradox of motherhood
is giving yourself to your child
so completely and deeply
while knowing that person
was never really yours to have.

A mother's love is truly
the most selfless love of all

I Promise

I am far from perfect
I am sensitive, complicated, anxious,
and a constant work in progress

I will make mistakes,
but I promise to always apologize and acknowledge my errors
I promise to be your constant in a world of variables
I promise to love you unconditionally and endlessly
I promise to offer you a safe space for your feelings, thoughts,
and concerns

I promise to always try my best,
although that varies day to day, hour to hour,
and even minute to minute
I promise to give you all my love, efforts, and guidance
I promise to walk beside you wherever life may take you
I promise to be your biggest cheerleader, supporter, and fan

I am full of flaws,
and I promise to never hide that from you
I promise you that it is safe to be imperfect
And I promise you that your heart is always safe with me

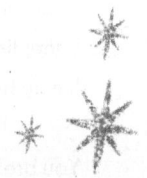

For the Mamas

Life can often seem like a game of whack-a-mole
We leap from one task to the next
We cross items off a list,
only to have more responsibilities pop up

The mental load is overwhelming, Mama.

Life feels like a mountain that we can never climb
And if we do climb it, we often lose our footing
And if we manage to keep our balance,
we have too much on our backs to reach the top

You're doing the best you can, Mama.

Life can feel exhausting
When they're babies, you're up all night with them
When they are sleeping through the night,
you stay up to accomplish things or to have time without kids
When you get into bed at a reasonable hour,
you stay up worrying and planning

It's okay to admit you need help, Mama.

Life can be painful
Sometimes it is for a brief period
Other times it lasts months or even years
It may be hard to remember a time when you weren't struggling

You are not alone with these feelings, Mama.

Life can spin you around and drop you in the middle of nowhere
Life can feel like you are constantly dealt the losing hand
Life can knock the wind out from under you
Life can make you unsure of left from right and up from down

You aren't meant to do it all, Mama.

Put the list down
Take the weight of the world off your shoulders
Hire a sitter
Go for a walk or read a book

Don't do it for your kids
Don't do it for your family
Don't do it for anyone else

Do it for you.

Because you need to take care of yourself.
Because your well-being is of the utmost importance.
Because you need to be your own friend.

It is time for you to love yourself, Mama.

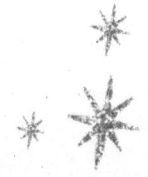

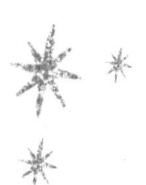

Mom Shaming

The mom shaming
needs to stop.

Moms second guess themselves
and feel enough guilt as it is.

We need to lift one another up
instead of tearing one another down.

I Would Do Anything for You

I would do anything for you.

I would face my greatest fears
I would shine a light on the parts of myself that I've hidden
I would shatter so I can properly fit the pieces of myself together

I would do anything for you.

I would allow exhaustion to eat away at me
I would crack myself open to the pain of letting you go
I would permanently sleep with one eye open

I would do anything for you.

I would lose parts of who I once was
I would stare at an unrecognizable reflection in the mirror
I would churn when I'm on empty

I would do anything for you.

I would prioritize you above myself
I would turn myself inside out to make you smile
I would stretch, scar, and tear my body

I would do anything for you.

I would fight for the strength to take care of you
I would speak up in situations where I feel uncomfortable
I would protect you at any cost

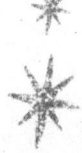

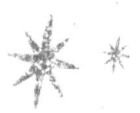

I would do anything for you.

I would hold my breath until I knew you were okay
I would advocate for what is best for you
I would permanently waltz with worry

I would do anything for you.

I would wait beside the phone to hear your voice
I would rearrange plans and schedules
I would educate myself to give you the necessary support

I would do anything for you.

I would let go of those who could cause you pain
I would work on myself every day
I would mold myself into what you need

I would do anything for you.

When you looked at me for the first time,
I looked deep into your eyes, and I knew.
I would do anything.

I would do anything for you.

Those Strong-Willed Children of Ours

Those strong-willed children of ours.

Their stubbornness and defiance.
How they overwhelm us
and push our buttons.

Although parenting is challenging,
we must remember not to break their spirit.
We must teach them to channel the flames
that burn so deeply within them.

Those strong-willed children of ours
will become strong-willed adults.

And their determination and resolve
will allow them to extinguish
injustices and cruelties that are thrown their way.

Those strong-willed children of ours
will blaze their own trail
instead of simply following it.

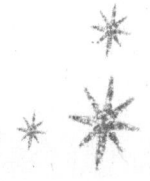

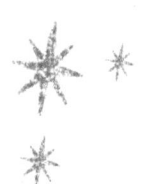

To the Mama Filled with Uncertainty

To the mama filled with uncertainty,
I see you trying
I see you doing your best
I see how you keep going
I see your heart

If you are consumed by doubt or guilt or exhaustion,
please remember...
you're doing great

Because everything you do,
you do out of love

Struggle

When our kids are struggling, we struggle too.

The kid at school who is struck with taunts and giggles.
The child who cannot focus on what the teacher is saying.
The classmate who eats alone at lunch.

Those kids have moms whose hearts bleed for them
every time they leave their home.

Children with feelings that aren't understood.
Children with needs that aren't met.
Children with voices that aren't heard.

Those children fight battles each day.
And their mothers do everything possible to arm them for battle.

We talk to teachers.
We have meetings.
We go to specialists.
We speak with other parents.

And we hope and pray that others will see the beautiful sparkle
that is our child.

Because although our children might sway to a different beat,
they are still playing the same drum.

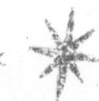

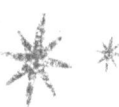

Our children struggle, and we shatter.
Bit by bit we pull ourselves apart trying to stop our children from unraveling.

And we hope and pray that others will see the magic that is our child.

Because when our kids struggle, we struggle too.

I Am a Flawed Mother

I am a flawed mother
I speak too much
I don't always listen
I rush to judgment
I react instead of respond.

I am a flawed mother,
but through the good times, the bad times, and the in-between,
I've always loved you
with all my heart.

I am a flawed mother,
but I will always stand by you
and support you
through the ebbs and flows of life.

I am a flawed mother,
but my love for you is unwavering
It is the one steady gift I can give you
in a world filled with chaos.

I am a flawed mother,
but I will always try my best
I will stumble and fall,
but I will continue to rise again.

I am a flawed mother,
but I am a mother who loves you
unconditionally and ferociously.
And that is what truly matters.

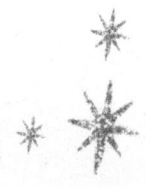

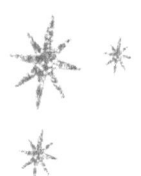

And I'm Grateful

Motherhood is overwhelming,
and I'm grateful to be a mom

Motherhood is tiring,
and I'm grateful to be a mom

Motherhood is stressful,
and I'm grateful to be a mom

Motherhood is filled with uncertainty,
and I'm grateful to be a mom

Acknowledging the difficulties of motherhood
doesn't mean we aren't grateful

Mom Guilt

Mom guilt is born alongside your child

it gnaws at your soul
eats away at your sense of self

Mom guilt feeds off your love

it makes you wonder if you're enough
it makes you feel your love isn't enough

Mom guilt is a parasite

it sucks away your semblance of self
it silently simmers and then boils over

Mom guilt is a hurricane

sweeping everything in its path
destroying you from the inside out

Mom guilt is sadistic

it wants you to suffer
it wants to make you feel shame

Mom guilt is a stalker

it finds you in your darkest hour
it silently simmers during your happiest moments

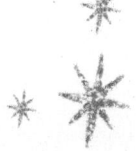

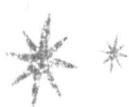

 Mom guilt doesn't discriminate

it doesn't matter your age, location, or religion
it doesn't matter your occupation or background

Mom guilt will destroy you

it will destroy everyone around you
if you allow it to consume you

So remind yourself that your love is what matters
Remind yourself that you're trying your best
Remind yourself that your best is what matters

Remember that your love is what your kids need
Remember that you are what they need
Remember that none of us are perfect

Mom guilt may sometimes win battles,
but it doesn't have to win the war

If you love unconditionally
and try your very best,
you are a good mom.

What We Model

I'm forgiving myself for my mistakes,
because I want my child to forgive herself.

I'm open with my emotions,
so my child is open with hers.

I'm loving myself unconditionally,
so my child loves herself unconditionally.

I'm prioritizing my inner beauty over my looks,
so my child knows that is what's most important.

I'm admitting when I'm wrong,
so that my child owns up to her own errors.

I'm striving for effort over perfection,
so my child knows that perfection is an illusion.

I'm showing myself kindness,
so my child treats herself with kindness.

I'm setting boundaries with others,
so my child knows how to set boundaries with others.

I'm practicing regulating my emotions,
so my child knows how to regulate hers.

What we model for our kids sets them up for how
they view themselves and the world.

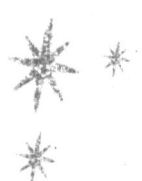

We Feel Everything

Motherhood brings the highest highs
and the lowest lows

Our children's happiness gives us bliss and
their sadness causes us depths of sorrows

We feel everything because
we love them so deeply and completely

And we always will

Moms Are Tired

Moms are tired.

from the endless demands
from the expectations of others
from the expectations we put on ourselves

Moms are tired.

from fatigue in our weary bones
from distress in our weary hearts
from inner chatter in our weary minds

Moms are tired.

from lullabies and illnesses
from endless to-do lists
from knowing everyone's schedules

Moms are tired.

from lack of sleep
from endless guilt
from comparisons to others

Moms are tired.

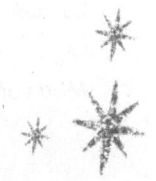

from the mental load
from the mom shaming
from the need to be everything to everyone

Moms are tired.

from running errands
from planning events
from remembering everything for everyone

Moms are tired.

from questioning our choices
from regretting our mistakes
from being everyone's source of comfort

Moms are tired.

an exhaustion that permeates our pores
an exhaustion that sleep cannot mend
an exhaustion that cranks and roars

Moms are tired.

because we need support
because we need understanding
because we need appreciation

Moms are tired.

because we love so deeply
because we give so willingly
because we start and end with our children

Moms are tired.

So tell a mother that she's a good mom.
So offer a mother assistance.
So voice your love and gratitude for her.

Because moms are always tired.

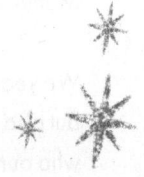

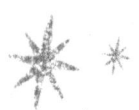

Motherhood Is Filled with Contradictions

Motherhood is filled with contradictions.

It causes us constant guilt,
while bringing us infinite joy
It is filled with uncertainty and fear,
while also showing us
a strength and courage within ourselves
that we didn't know existed.

Kids will push our buttons and
test our patience more than anyone else,
but we would walk through fire for them
without a moment's hesitation.

We feel overwhelmed and crave time to ourselves,
but we feel sad
and like a part of us is missing
when they aren't around.

It is the hardest thing we'll ever do,
but loving our kids is the easiest thing we'll ever do.

Motherhood is filled with contradictions.

We yearn for the previous versions of our kids,
but also love and cherish
who our kids are in the present.

It is the greatest responsibility of our lives,
as well as the greatest privilege
We teach and guide our kids,
but our kids are our greatest teachers of all.

It robs us of our own identity,
while molding us into a better version of ourselves
It is filled with messiness, chaos, and unpredictability,
as well as tenderness, love, and beauty.

Motherhood is filled with contradictions.

It will bring us our highest highs and lowest lows.

Motherhood is filled with contradictions.

But the love...
a mother's love.

That love is constant.

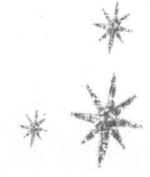

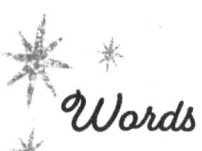
Words

The saying is that words don't hurt
but they do

Words can build people up
or tear them down

Words can make someone's day
feel brighter or darker

Words can be a new perspective
or a trigger

Words do matter

Let's use words to show
kindness
grace
and compassion

And let's teach our kids
to do the same

Mistakes

No matter how much
we love our children
we are always going
to make mistakes

What works for one child
may not work for another child
What works one time
may not work the next time

Children don't come with
instruction manuals
Give yourself grace

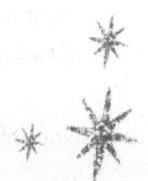

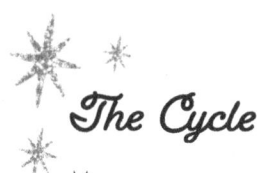

The Cycle

Moms compare.

We compare ourselves to other moms.
We compare because we don't feel like we measure up.
We feel bad about ourselves,
which causes us to compare,
which causes us to feel even worse.

It is a vicious cycle of comparison and guilt.

Everywhere we turn we feel we are falling short.
The mom at carpool who always looks like she stepped out of a magazine.
The women on social media with the seamless marriages,
the endless friends,
and the impeccable homes.

Perfection constantly rings in our ears,
but we are unable to sing the tune.

How do they do it?
Why can't we do it?

The truth is,
we all have different lives,
but we aren't all that different.

None of us have it all together.

You don't know what's really going on inside that mom
who makes you feel inadequate.
You don't know the pressure she feels every morning to look
and act a certain way.
You don't know the struggles she goes through.

But I promise you,
she has her own hardships too.

We don't know what goes on behind closed doors.
If that perfect couple hasn't shared a bed in the last five years.
If that perfect house is the result of a spouse
who is always working to afford it.
If that woman with countless friends
has never had a genuine conversation with them
about how much her heart aches and how stressed she feels.

We all have our own unique set of circumstances,
but at our core we aren't really all that different.

We all feel.
We all worry,
and cry,
and doubt,
and love,
and care,
and hurt,
and feel unsure.

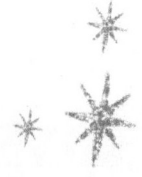

Trials and Tribulations of Motherhood

We need to stop comparing ourselves.
Because we are all human.
Because we are doing the best we can
with the cards we were dealt.

Let's stop the perpetual cycle of comparison and guilt.

Let's stop comparing.
Because nobody is perfect.

You are enough.
I am enough.

We are enough.

I Am a Mother Who Is Exhausted

I am a mother who is exhausted.

My exhaustion has seeped into every pore,
into every muscle,
into every fiber of my being.

Yet I cannot sleep.
There are too many thoughts running through my mind.
No matter how much my body shuts down,
my mind cannot shut down with it.

My thoughts wander as I lie awake.

I think about the look on my daughter's face when I scolded her.
I think about the endless things I need to do.
It feels like no matter how much I try to accomplish,
there is always something else.
I think about all the ways I should have done better,
could have done better.

Although I am exhausted, I cannot sleep.

Instead, I run the to-do list through my head.
Did I pay all the bills?
The backyard is a disaster.
When is the dishwasher repair man coming again?

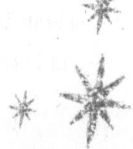

Did I read enough books to my daughter today?
I cleaned the house; why does it still look like a mess?
Was she dressed warmly enough when I let her play outside?

The biggest question that pokes at my brain and my heart—
does my daughter know how much I love her?

With all the responsibilities, all the stress, all the juggling,
does she know that being her mom is what is most important?

I tell her, but does she understand
when she is too young to grasp all of life's pressures?

Does she see that I try to give so much,
but there is only one of me to give?

I am a mother who is exhausted.

Exhausted from caring.
From trying.
From putting one foot in front of the other
when I can't always see clearly where I'm trying to go.

I am a mother who is exhausted but cannot sleep.

Instead, I tiptoe into my daughter's room,
and I watch her sleep.
I watch her sleep,
and I know she feels completely and deeply loved.

As I watch her,
I remember that every struggle is worth it
because of that little girl sleeping peacefully.

I will always worry,
I will always have concerns,
and I will always feel that I'm doing it all wrong.

I will always be exhausted.

That's because I'm a mother.

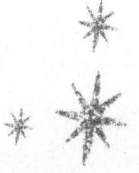

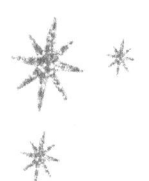

The Storm

The sun peeks through the clouds
even at the darkest times of motherhood
You will recall it vividly
but it is impossible to bask in it whilst it storms

Let the rain wash away your pain
and remember that it is always darkest before dawn
The sun will shine again

I Pray You'll Remember

What kind of mother will you see
when you look at me?
What kind of impact will I have on you
when you are older?

I pray you'll remember a mother
who owned up to her errors.
Who was rough around the edges,
but always tried to smooth them out.

I pray you'll remember a mother
who would assuage your fears.
A mother who was always there for you.
A mother who prioritized you.

I pray you'll remember a mother
who practiced what she preached.
Who showed kindness to others.
Who tried to give kindness to herself.

I pray you'll remember a mother
who lit up when she saw you.
Whose arms were your safe place.
Who gave you advice and let you vent.

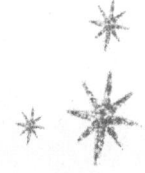

I pray you'll remember a mother
who was present physically and emotionally.
A mother you look up to.
A mother you appreciate.

I pray you'll remember a mother
whose morals you admire.
A woman who is your role model.
A woman who never gave up.

I pray you'll remember a mother
with whom you shared countless happy memories.
I pray your eyes will always twinkle
when you say, "That's my mother."

Listen to Your Heart

Listen to your heart
when you're consumed by regret and self-doubt.

Listen to your heart
when the pieces of yourself don't quite fit together.

Listen to your heart
when you question your self-worth.

Listen to your heart
when words of fire erupt from your lips.

Listen to your heart
when waves of guilt encapsulate your very being.

Listen to your heart
when you feel like you never measure up.

Listen to your heart
when your inner critic echoes in your mind.

Listen to your heart
when the mistakes you've made are playing on an endless loop.

Listen to your heart
when loneliness pierces your heart.

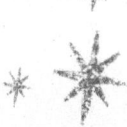

Listen to your heart
when you don't recognize your reflection in the mirror.

Listen to your heart
when fear is your constant companion.

Listen to your heart,
and you will always find your way back home.

Listen to your heart.

Imperfect

Mothers are imperfect,
but their unconditional love for their children
is exactly as it should be

And that makes them perfect
in the eyes of their children.

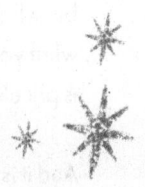

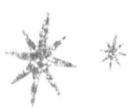

The Demands of Motherhood Are High

The demands of motherhood are high.

The exhaustion.
The overwhelm.
The frustration.
The guilt.

There are times when I can barely catch my breath.
There are times when I don't know left from right
and up from down.

And in those moments, I stop.
I stop and think of you, my child.

I hear your laughter.
I feel your embrace.
I look at your smile.

And it lifts me up.
It lights me up.

The demands of motherhood are high,
but what it gives me—
what you give me—
is priceless.

And it is worth it in infinite ways every single day.

Motherhood Is Hard

Motherhood is amazing, a blessing,
and the most rewarding thing I've ever done.
It is also the biggest responsibility and the most difficult thing
I've ever done.

The fact of the matter is,
motherhood is hard.

Admitting that doesn't mean I'm not grateful to be a mom;
there isn't a single day that I don't feel gratitude.
Declaring that doesn't mean that I don't feel honored
to be a mom;
I know what a privilege it is.
Accepting that doesn't mean that I don't love my daughter;
I love her with every ounce of my being.

Motherhood is hard. Period.

We can acknowledge the feelings of overwhelm, exhaustion,
and frustration,
without always having to acknowledge how wondrous it is.
We need to be open and honest
about the messiness of motherhood,
without feeling guilt or shame.

Because the reality is that motherhood is hard.

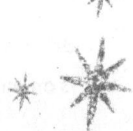

Trials and Tribulations of Motherhood

If you are having a bad day, week, or season of motherhood,
that is okay.
If you are not savoring every minute of motherhood,
that is okay.
If you are counting down the hours until bedtime,
that is okay.
If you miss the days of life before kids,
that is okay.
If you put your kid on the iPad or in front of the TV
so you could get a break,
that is okay.
That doesn't make us bad moms.
It makes us human.

Let's discuss the struggles of motherhood,
without feeling the need to add positivity.

Because when we are honest about how hard it is,
that takes some of the weight off our already
overburdened shoulders.
It allows us to simply feel how we are feeling
so we can get through it.
It allows us to come out the other side,
so we can dust ourselves off, straighten ourselves up,
and be better moms to our kids.

Motherhood is hard.

Because taking care of another human being
is an enormous responsibility.

Motherhood is incredibly hard.
And sometimes, we can just leave it at that.

Outer Beauty

Outer beauty is something that changes
with the sands of time
Inner beauty is an investment
that lasts a lifetime

Let's raise our children to focus on the
type of beauty that truly matters

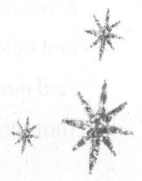

Just

"Just" is often attached to the hip
of the word "mother."
I am just a mother.

A way of diminishing
our own efforts.
A way of dismissing
our greatest role.

Just a mother
implies trivialization.
Just a mother
implies minimization.

The words "just" and "mother" are like oil and water.
For what we do is crucial.
What we do is irreplaceable.
What we are is meaningful.

You are not just a mother.
You are so much more than a word.
You embody love.
You embody eternity.

Mothers are the glue
that hold their families together.
And that should never be forgotten.
That should never be minimized.

You are everything to your children.
Because you are their mother.

How Deeply She Is Loved

When harsh words escape my mouth
and frustration blinds my vision,
I pray she knows how deeply she is loved.

When I'm scrambling through night's activities
and cannot beat the ticking of the clock,
I pray she knows how deeply she is loved.

When I'm battling my own struggles
and my inner tank is churning on low,
I pray she knows how deeply she is loved.

When her heart shatters into pieces
and I'm unable to ease her pain,
I pray she knows how deeply she is loved.

Although the words are looped through her brain
I want their meaning to be as engrained as the air she breathes
I want her to grasp with the utmost certainty
that she was and always will be deeply loved.

There are no words or actions that can diminish it,
because a mother's love has no bounds or limits
In her darkest hour and brightest moments
I pray she knows how deeply she is loved.

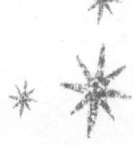

And when she gets older and has children of her own
I hope she will look at them, smile, and say,
"Now I finally understand it all.
I know how deeply I was loved."

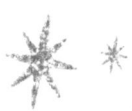

I Was Chosen to Be Your Mom

I was chosen to be your mom.

When I'm tired,
I remember that I was chosen
and I pull myself out of bed

When I'm frustrated,
I remember that I was chosen
and I try to be more patient

When I feel down,
I remember that I was chosen
and I pick myself back up

I make many mistakes,
and I don't have all the answers,
but there isn't a moment that I don't feel blessed

Because I was chosen to be your mom.

Polar Feelings

Being a mother means juggling emotions.
Emotions that seem impossible to contain at once.

Yet it is those polar feelings
that encapsulate the essence of motherhood.

You can feel grateful you're a mother
and not love every moment of it.

You can love your kids with all of your heart
and feel anger for the buttons they push.

You can yearn for moments of solitude from your children
yet ache when you are apart from them.

You can want to rewind the moments of contentment
while wanting to fast forward the moments of struggle.

You can dislike a behavior or choice,
while liking who they are as a person.

You can miss prior versions of them,
while opening your arms to who they are now.

You can feel unlucky about life circumstances,
while feeling lucky to be a mother.

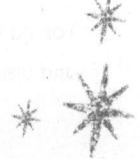

You can acknowledge the hardships of motherhood
while understanding that motherhood is a blessing.

You can encourage them to spread their wings,
while knowing their absence will break your heart.

You can want to shelter them from life's pain
while accepting that storms are inevitable.

You can close the door on who you were
while opening a window on who you're becoming.

You can allow them to fall down
even though your instinct is to hold them up.

You can support their life choices
while knowing you'd choose differently.

You can feel every ounce of joy they bring
and feel every ounce of pain they cause.

You can love them with all of your heart
and feel lost with all of your soul.

You can grieve your life before motherhood
while other pieces of you come to life.

You can feel exhaustion in every fiber
and discover inner strength runs through your veins.

You can be their greatest teacher
while being their greatest student.

You can think you have all the answers
and find yourself with a new set of questions.

You can feel like you are lacking direction
while discovering your greatest purpose.

You can wear many hats in life,
but be unable to wear them all at once.

You can give them all of you
and know they are never fully yours to have.

You can feel life knocked you over
only to realize the right way to stand up.

Allow yourself to feel the fangs of life
to prevent them from swallowing you whole.

For it is those polar feelings
that contain motherhood's deepest meaning.

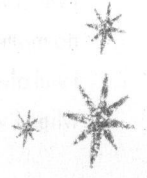

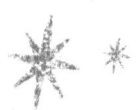

I Am Human.
I Am a Mother.

From the moment you were born,
I've made mistakes
Despite my best intentions,
I mess up over and over again
No matter how much I love you,
I will never get it all right

I am human.

From the moment you were born,
you have seen me frazzled
You have seen me overwhelmed more times than I can count
You have seen me frustrated when I should have been
more patient
You have seen me speak when I should have listened
You have seen me uncertain and second-guessing my choices

I am human.

From the moment you were born,
I have loved you with every ounce of my being
I will always try to do right by you
I will always get back up,
no matter how many times I may fall down
I will always apologize to you
when I've done something wrong

I will always put one foot in front of the other,
no matter my uncertainty

I will never get it all right,
but I will always keep trying

I am a mother.

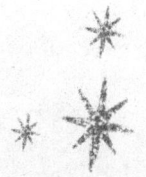

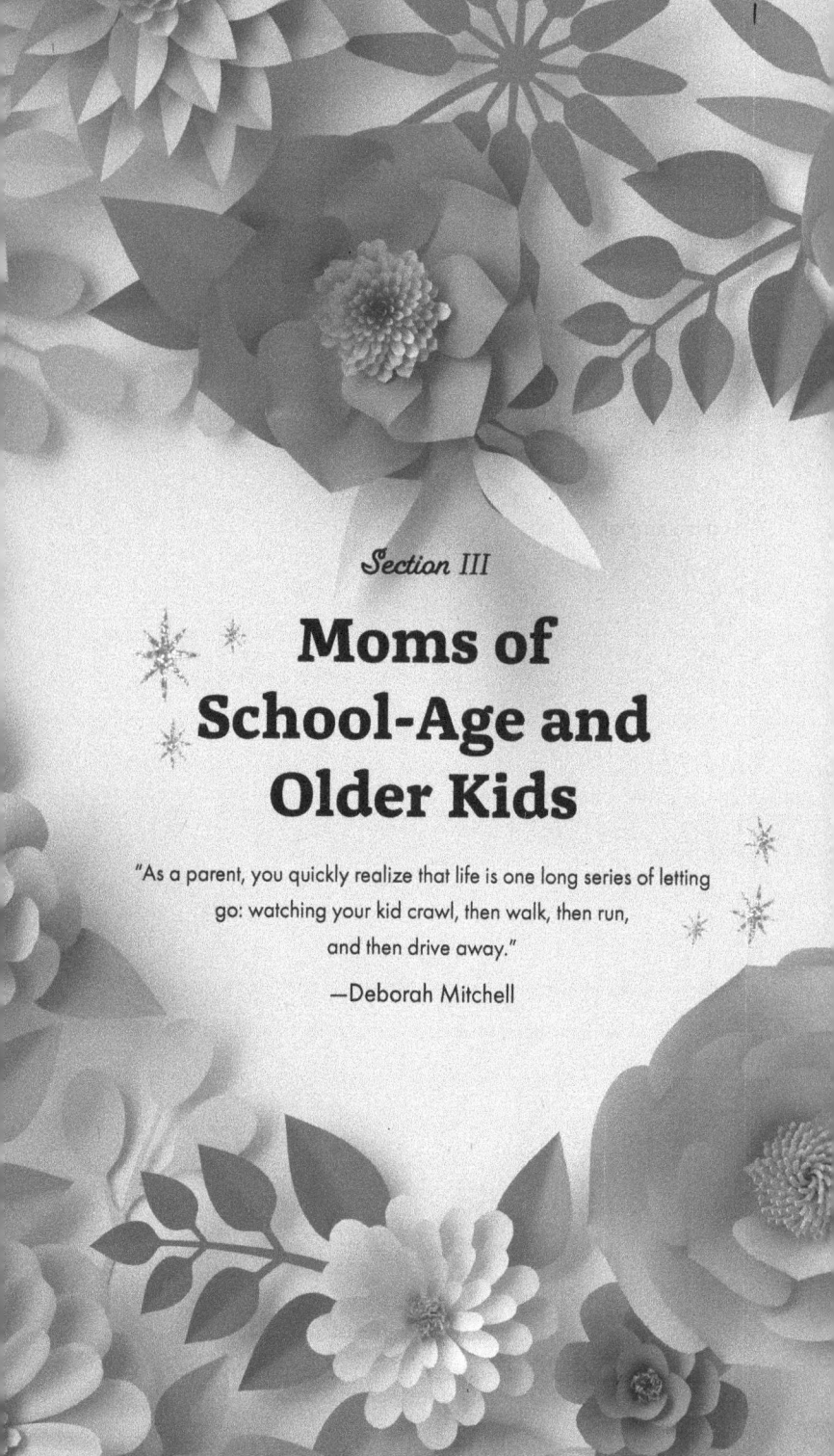

Section III

Moms of School-Age and Older Kids

"As a parent, you quickly realize that life is one long series of letting go: watching your kid crawl, then walk, then run, and then drive away."

—Deborah Mitchell

A Stolen Heart

There once was a baby
who stole my heart.

When she was placed in my arms,
I felt the immediate need to protect her
I would stare at her
and the world stopped when she smiled

There once was a toddler
who stole my heart.

She would fall,
and fear cascaded down my spine
She would run,
while I prayed she'd forever run into my arms

There once was a young child
who stole my heart.

She found wonder and beauty
in all that surrounded her
And every single time she laughed,
the sky sparkled and the sun shone a bit brighter

There once was a child
who stole my heart.

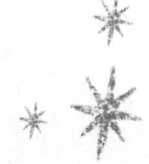

Her strong will was only surpassed by her sensitivity
She did things her own way,
in her own time,
and I was consumed by equal parts frustration and awe

There once was a young lady
who stole my heart.

I saw reminders of every version of her
that I had known and loved
while glimpses of who she'd become intensified
And when she laughed and smiled,
light still peeked its way into every blackened corner

There once was a being, ever growing,
who stole my heart.

For when life was blown into her soul
my heart was placed there alongside it.

You Will Always Be My Baby

You're not a baby anymore,
but you will always be my baby.

I want to turn back time
so I can cradle you in my arms again.
I also want to savor every moment
of the child you are right now.

My precious one—
Do you know how much my heart breaks as I watch you grow?
Do you know how proud I am of the person you are becoming?

I want to cling to you,
but I also know the beauty of watching you soar.

You are finding yourself,
but I am finding myself too.

You are not a baby anymore,
but you will always be my baby.

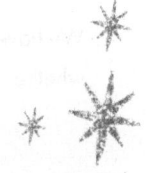

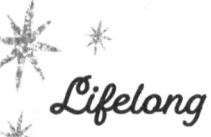

Lifelong

"We only have eighteen summers with our children"
is the phrase drummed into our heads.

"Enjoy it while you can"
is the message stamped upon our minds.

"It only gets harder"
are the words etched into our hearts.

The pressure on mothers to savor the moment
while being mindful of an expiration date
causes endless cycles of guilt and worry.

And although life changes
as our children transform before our eyes,
it does not mean that our life with them is over.

Our role as mothers does not end.
It is reshaped as our children grow.
It ebbs and flows, waxes and wanes.

It shifts and bends,
but it is never broken
for our connection to our children is never severed.

We have a lifelong commitment to our children
whether they are eighteen months or forty-eight years.

The path to our hearts
must always be open and available.

The trying and effort
continues for the course of our lives.
The unconditional love we have for our children
is everlasting and does not expire.

And although we may miss prior versions
and think fondly upon their younger years,
some things will never change.

We are always mothers,
and our commitment to our children is lifelong.

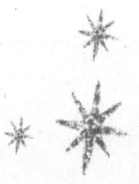

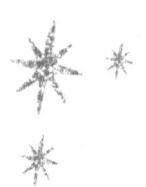

Every Moment

I haven't loved
every
moment
of
motherhood,
but I've loved
every
moment
of being your mom

Holding On

I know I have to let you go as you get older,
but I'm focusing on holding on.

Holding on to being your biggest fan and cheerleader
Holding on to the warmth of your smile
and the sound of your laughter
Holding on to feeling so deeply, no matter your age
Holding on to how grateful I am to be your mom

Holding on to the twinkle in your eyes
when I tell you that I love you
Holding on to the promise that I will always offer you guidance,
advice, and support
Holding on to carrying you in my heart, wherever you may go
Holding on to the beauty of the past, the gift of the present,
and the joy of the future

Holding on to the feeling of your head
gently resting on my shoulder
Holding on to the unconditional love
between a mother and a child
Holding on to the privilege of raising an amazing person
Holding on to the reality that letting you go doesn't mean
that I can't hold on to all of these things

So I can let go.
But know I will always be there holding on.

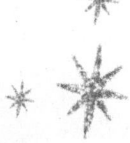

She Is My Daughter

She finds the wonder in everything
She smiles and the world feels a bit brighter
She jumps first and asks questions later
She is my student and my greatest teacher

She is the reason I worry,
and the reason my heart overflows with love
She tests limits and challenges me daily
She loves deeply and cares fiercely
She marches to the beat of her own drum

She lights up my life in every way
She is the reason I am irrevocably changed

She is my daughter.

The Flower

A tiny seed is planted,
and sprinkled with love.
After months of waiting,
its roots are firmly planted.

The sun crests its golden head,
and kisses are planted upon its stem.
Drops of dew and hope
shower the parched ground.

As the growing seedling leaves its mark
upon the unsteady world,
tears of equal parts joy and sorrow
cascade from every corner.

When the wind whirls
and the storms howl,
gentle whispers and still waters
provide shelter and steady land.

The plant begins to grow
for its beauty cannot be contained.
And it radiates like the sun
that shines firmly upon it.

The flower now stands tall.
Bloomed petals proud and vibrant.

But that flower will always remember
the rain and iridescent sun
that encouraged it to sparkle.

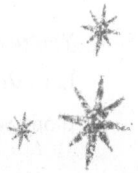

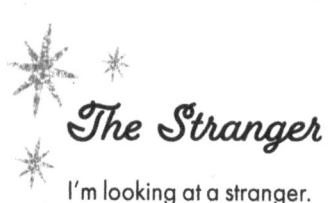

The Stranger

I'm looking at a stranger.

The back talking.
The hands on your hips.
The eye-rolling.
The moodiness.
The pushing me away.

You're no longer a little child,
but not an adult.

Each day I feel like I am struggling to comprehend a new world
without knowing any of the rules.
I feel helpless.
I know you're trying to find yourself,
but I am trying to find you too.

Then I look into your eyes,
and I see the same eyes I've stared into since you were born.
I watch you sleep,
and I see the same innocence
strewn across the shadows of your face.
I see you smile or hear you humming,
and I get reminders that you are still you.

You're evolving into an older version of yourself,
but you're taking the intricacies of who you were
along with you.

You're trying to navigate the world
in this new in-between phase of your life,
and there will be many hiccups along the way.

You're not alone, my in-between child.
I'm right here with you.

Although I have to step back a bit
and let you find your own way,
never forget I am there with open arms and an open heart.

As you forge your own path,
know I'll be watching and traveling along with you.

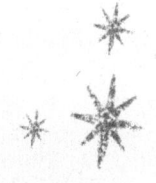

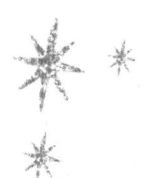

Sweet Child

Sweet Child,

I don't have all of life's answers,
but I know this to be true...

No matter where you go,
no matter what you do,
a part of you
will always be with me,
and a part of me
will always be with you.

Love,
Mom

I Look at You

I look at you,
and I see your eyelashes fluttering as I rock you to sleep,
I hear the sounds of laughter as we played peek-a-boo,
I reimagine the widening of your eyes as you took in
every object, every person, every sound.

I look at you,
and I see your tiny feet scampering across the floor,
you stretching your arms to ask me to carry you,
you squealing with delight as you chased bubbles
and spun in circles.

I look at you,
and I see you slowly sounding out words on my lap,
how your backpack overpowered your tiny frame,
your eyes narrowing in concentration
as you practiced tying your shoes,
your little legs pumping on the swings,
your face lighting up as I'd hold you in my arms
and dance around the room.

I look at you,
and I see you reading chapter books on your bed,
putting your arm through mine as we take walks,
your brow furrowing as you help me bake,
your head resting on my shoulder as we listen to music,
your chuckles as you tell me a joke.

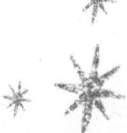

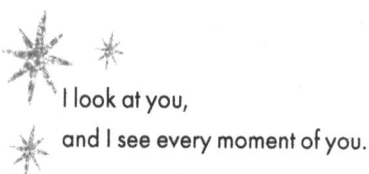
I look at you,
and I see every moment of you.

The echoes of the past,
the calling of the present,
and the gentle whispers of what will come.

I see my baby,
my little girl,
and my not-so-little girl
all in front of me.

I look at you,
and I see everything.

And I am so grateful for all of it.

I Am a Mom Who Always Says, "I Love You"

I am a mom who always says, "I love you."

In moments of comfort and sorrow,
"I love you" is often said amidst a big hug
"I love you" are the last words you hear before you go to sleep
When we aren't seeing eye to eye, "I love you" interrupts
exasperated words and angry silences

I am a mom who always says, "I love you."

Times of celebration aren't complete without an "I love you"
Moments of guilt and apologies
will always be followed by "I love you"
"I love you" is written on notes and cards and slipped under
your bedroom door

I am a mom who always says, "I love you."

I say it with and without cause, with and without response
I say it because those three simple words carry
immeasurable meaning
I say it because I want it to cling to the air you breathe

I am a mom who always says, "I love you."

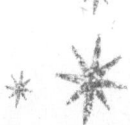

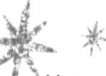

You might tire of hearing it
You might roll your eyes when I say it,
but you will never, ever question it

Because I am a mom who will always say, "I love you."

Not Everyone

My Child,

Not everyone
is going to like you,
and that is okay

It isn't your job
to get others
to like you

It is your job to like yourself

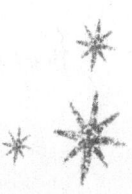

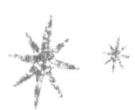

There Is Not Just One Kind of Smart

Every child is smart.
Book smarts measure one intelligence.
But there are many others.

There are kids who are brilliant with their empathy and kindness.
Some kids excel at spatial relations.
Other kids are gifted at communicating
with everyone around them.

There is not just one kind of smart.

The kid that struggles in school may be an amazing artist.
The kid that sits by himself might be a whiz on the computer.
The kid that is terrible at math might shine as a writer.

There is not just one kind of smart.

Some kids are great at public speaking.
Some kids are awkward around people
but are comfortable with animals.
Some kids are poor test takers,
and their academic intelligence cannot be accurately measured.

There is not just one kind of smart.

When we emphasize one form of intelligence,
it dismisses the importance of the other ways they glow.
Each kid has their own inner spark.
And we can encourage them to do their best in all areas,
while ensuring that their flame never extinguishes.

Because when we remember
that there isn't just one kind of smart,
we appreciate the beauty of all types of embers.

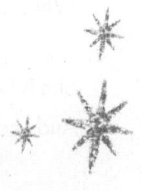

She Is Her Own Person

My child might look like me
My child might say things that resemble what I say

But she is her own person.

The world doesn't need another me,
and I wouldn't want her to be me

She is her own person.

A person with tracings and intricacies
with illuminations and motifs
that are completely hers

Some things may be harder for her,
but there are things that come to her seamlessly
her love of meeting new people
her ability to live in the moment
her fearlessness and zest for life

The world doesn't need another me
It needs her, just as she is

Whatever roads she may choose
Whatever path she may forge

She is her own person.
And I couldn't be prouder.

Grieve

I watched recordings of my child.
As the images flashed before my eyes,
I realized I knew them all.
I felt the thoughts, feelings, and circumstances,
as if they had just occurred.
Although they had long passed,
those cascading images were forever etched in my mind.

They were the tapestries of my soul,
the pages of my heart.
They might wither at the edges,
or yellow with the passage of time,
but they could never be reduced to ash.
The binding would never break,
for it was stitched together with love.

I watched her cry, laugh, and smile,
and I felt it all.
My heart shattered into pieces
while simultaneously reconstructing itself.
It filled me with hope,
alongside pain that brought me to my knees.

I saw the playback of every memory
and heard an echo
that was both far away and close by.
It was a calling that reverberated both forward and backwards.

I grieve the child she was at every age,
for she will never be that age again.
I yearn to feel her little hands
rest softly on my cheek.
To take in the scent of the top of her head
that smelled like youth.

I have lost all that she once was,
while gaining all that she is now.
The heartbreak and heart bursts
of every passage of time
are filled with despair and gratitude.
A yearning for what was, is,
and what is yet to come.

We feel contradictory feelings all at once,
and all with such intensity.
For mothers carry within us
the greatest contradiction of all.
We ache for the previous forms of our children,
and cherish exactly who our children are right now.

My World

You are my north star
an anchor when I've lost my way

You are my sun
lighting up even my darkest days

You are my moon
a pull that's felt deep within me

Child, you are my world,
and my world you always will be

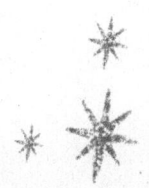

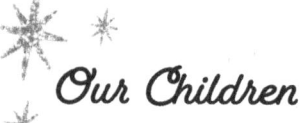

Our Children

Whenever our children leave,
a piece of our hearts leaves with them.

Whether they are going to school
or leaving the nest,
a part of us is missing.

Whenever cruel words are spoken to our children,
it feels like daggers to our heart.
We want to protect them from the world.
We want to shelter them from life's storms.

Whenever our children feel helpless,
we feel a sense of panic
that makes it hard to breathe.

We want to take away their pain.
We want to make sure they are safe.
We want to fill them with confidence and love.

Whatever our children feel
a mother feels, too.
Because our hearts, minds, and prayers
are always with our children.

Kids Remember

Kids remember who shows up.

They remember
who cheers for them at their games

They remember
who spends time with them

They remember
who they go to for guidance and support

Gifts and toys are remembered temporarily

Love is remembered forever.

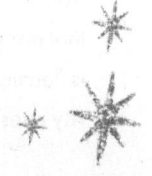

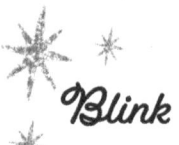

Blink

They say, "Blink and you'll miss it."
But I never blinked.
I saw it all.

I was there for every step, word, and performance.
I was there for every mishap, scrape, and scuffle.

But when I look back
to when my world turned
from black and white
to swirls of color,
there were times when my eyes
yearned to shut.

My eyes yearned to close
from the exhaustion that lay
deep within my bones.
My eyes yearned to shut
for a moment of solitude and silence.
My eyes yearned to close
from my body being touched,
pressed, pulled, and prodded.

My eyes yearned to shut
from the weight of reminders
that early motherhood
is fleeting and precious.
My eyes yearned to close

from the knowledge that time passed
would echo in my mind and my heart.

When I look back upon those early years,
I didn't miss a moment,
and there are things I do not miss.

But when there's stillness in the air,
the taunting in my ear
says that I am but a few chapters
in the story of my child's life.

Once upon a time I was the sun,
and she would orbit around me.
Once upon a time I was the moon,
and she was the tide.

It was a time when my kiss made the pain go away
and my arms wronged every right.
When gentle whispers and words of love
made all of life's monsters wither.
When a smile and caress
could soothe every sorrow.

It's okay to blink,
for there's much I do not miss.
But she will forever be my world,
yet she was never mine to have.

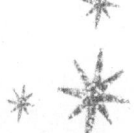

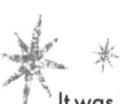

It was but a moment
that I was hers and she was mine.
It was but a moment
that I will carry forever in my heart.

That time is what I crave.
That time is what I cherish.

That blessing filled my lungs with air
and beat hope within my heart.
It's okay to blink,
but I will miss that until I breathe my last breath.

More Like You

I sometimes can't help
but stare at you

your enthusiasm
your confidence
your fierceness
your authenticity
your courage

I know I'm supposed to be your role model,
but I want to be more like you

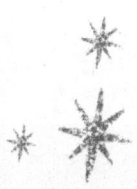

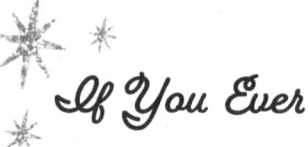
If You Ever

If you ever feel afraid,
remember you are brave

If you ever feel unloved,
remember you are loved beyond measure

If you ever feel lost,
remember you always have a home

If you ever feel unsure,
remember to listen to your inner voice

If you ever feel like giving up,
remember you are capable

If you ever hear words of cruelty or disrespect,
remember your strength and worth

If you ever feel life trying to crush you,
remember how high you are meant to soar

If you ever feel alone,
remember I am always with you

We May

We may tuck our children into their beds for a short time,
but we will always breathe a sigh of relief
when they get home safely

We may carry our children in our arms for a short time,
but we will always carry our children in our hearts

We may kiss our children's scrapes
and wipe their tears for a short time,
but we will always feel their pain

We may be our children's worlds for a short time,
but they will be ours for a lifetime

No matter their age,
we are always connected to our children through love

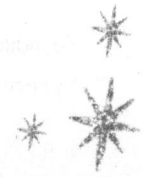

No

In a world filled with pressure and temptation,
it is important for our children to unflinchingly say "no."

Say no to the stranger who is asking you to come closer.
Say no to the popular kid who wants you to pull a prank.
Say no to the friend who encourages you to skip school.

It is okay to say no.

Say no to the partner who wants you
to do anything before you're ready.
Say no to pants that don't fit you
or make you feel badly about yourself.
Say no to the voice in your head
that whispers you aren't enough.

It is important to say no.

Say no to anyone who questions your worth.
Say no to anyone who doesn't respect you.
Say no to anything that makes you feel uncomfortable.

They must learn to say no to us,
if we project our own desires and dreams onto our children.

No matter where it is coming from,
it is necessary to say no.

We can teach our kids to be kind,
while standing up for themselves.
We can teach our kids to care for others,
while always caring for themselves.
We can show them that self-respect
sometimes means walking away.

When the voices of others are ringing in their ears,
their voice needs to be the one they hear first and foremost.

Because there is so much power in saying no.

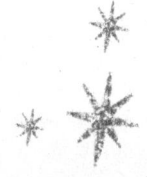

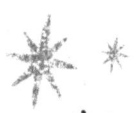

You Are Beautiful in Every Way

My child,
Take these words with you always—
You are beautiful in every way.

The kind of beauty that radiates from within
The kind of beauty that permeates your laugh and smile
The kind of beauty embodied in all that you do
The kind of beauty that is everlasting

And when the world is cold and cruel
I pray you always know these words to be true
For you are beautiful in every way.

Bind It

The pages of your life will turn,
but my love will always bind it.

Carry that love with you wherever you may go.
Carry that love with you when you are filled with doubts.
Carry that love with you when you question others.
Carry that love with you when you question yourself.

You may feel like the world is spinning,
but I pray my love anchors you.
You may feel like the world is cruel,
but I pray my love comforts you.

My love for you is constant.
My love for you is unconditional.
My love for you is forever.

Although the pages of your life will turn,
my love will always bind it.

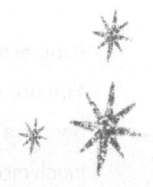

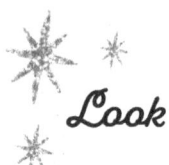

Look

Look for the hug where they squeeze extra tightly
Look for the giggles that cannot be contained
Look for the gaze that searches for yours
across a crowded room

Look for the whispered "I love you"
Look for the chatter
about seemingly nothing
and everything all at once

Look for the mere moments
of lingering by your side
Look at how their body relaxes
when you offer comfort and reassurance

Look for the twinkle in their eyes
when you tell them that you love them
Look for the smile on their lips
when you tell them you are proud

Just look
and you'll see
that your love
is what they need

Look at how you are what they need
You are who they'll always need
because you're getting it right
much more than you think

Look.
Look.
Just look.

And you'll see love.

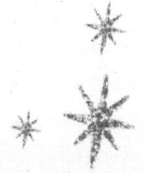

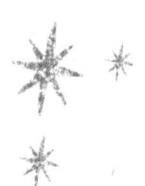

Leave the Nest

One day my child
will leave the nest

It is my job to teach her
how to spread her wings
while showing her
I will always be there
with open arms
if she should fall

Infinite Ways

A mother's love shows up in infinite ways.

When she listens by the doorway
to hear her child's gentle breathing
When she reads stories and sings for hours
When her child's pain causes her pain,
and her child's happiness causes her sheer bliss

A mother's love shows up in infinite ways.

When her heart both breaks and bursts at every first
When she lets go as her child becomes more independent,
even though all she wants is to keep them close
When she offers a shoulder to cry on, an ear to listen,
and arms to wrap around them in comfort

A mother's love shows up in infinite ways.

When she misses her child when they are not around
When she second guesses her choices and is filled with guilt
When she prays that her child knows the depth of her love

A mother's love shows up in infinite ways.

When she gives her all
regardless of what life has thrown her way
When she guides, supports, helps with homework,
and takes her kids to activities
When she is their biggest cheerleader and number one fan

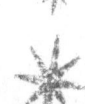

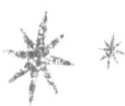

 A mother's love shows up in infinite ways.

When she sends messages to check on them
When she counts down the moments
until she can hug them again
When she worries about them, no matter their age

Children grow older
Life changes
But a mother's love?

That will always show up in infinite ways.

The Ache

The ache for the soft skin
that lay across my chest
The ache for high-pitched giggles
and toothless grins

The ache for the pitter patter
of tiny footsteps down the stairs
The ache for hands that reached for mine
and scribbles hung on the fridge

The ache to be your compass
and source of gravity in this world
The ache for innocence
and doing mundane things that are everything

The ache of guilt
for what resides within my mind
The ache of loss
for what I carried within my body
The ache of love
for what lies within my heart

The ache that entangles me with you.

The ache that throbs for eternity.

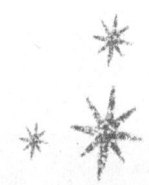

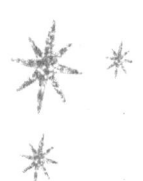

Power of Voices

Let's raise our children to
express their feelings openly
Let's teach our children that
true strength is found in kindness,
empathy, and compassion

Let's raise our children
to speak their minds
Let's teach our children
to stand up for themselves and others

Let's show our children the power
of their voices and their hearts

Constant

Motherhood is loving wholeheartedly,
trying,
falling down,
getting up,
and trying again.

Motherhood is loving completely,
feeling guilty,
praying they know how much they are loved,
and wondering what you could have done differently.

Motherhood is loving unconditionally,
frustration,
exhaustion,
second guessing yourself,
and all-consuming uncertainty.

But no matter our struggles,
the mistakes that are made,
or what stage of motherhood we are in,
motherhood is loving.

And a mother's love is constant.

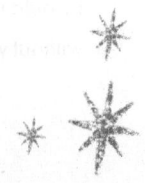

You Are My Greatest Teacher

Although I am the parent, you are my greatest teacher.

You taught me that there is no more beautiful sound
than the sound of your laughter.
You taught me that your hugs are worth more than any gift.
You taught me that it is okay to make mistakes.
You taught me that the love between a parent and a child
is unconditional.

You taught me that nothing I imagined could prepare me
for motherhood.
You taught me to slow down, enjoy the moment, and just be.
You taught me that I needed to learn to love myself
so I could teach you to love yourself.
You taught me that you don't need a perfect mom;
you need a mom who loves and supports you.

You taught me that being a parent requires endless patience
and coffee.
You taught me that it is possible
for your heart to explode with love.
You taught me to erase any notion I had
of what parenting is supposed to be.
You taught me that being a mother meant
I would never go to sleep again
without worrying and feeling guilty.

You taught me that motherhood is about thinking
you've got it all figured out,
only to realize you will always have new things to learn.
You taught me that the best moments in life
are the simplest ones—
snuggling with you, telling jokes, and holding your hand in mine.
You taught me that your smile is the best medicine in the world.
You taught me that motherhood is messy, hectic,
unpredictable, chaotic, and absolutely beautiful,
all rolled into one.

Most of all, you taught me that the gift of motherhood
is precious and priceless.
I will carry these lessons in my heart forever.

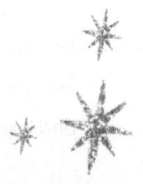

When You Think of Me

When you think of me,
I hope you will remember
rocking on your chair
as you nestled in my arms.

When you think of me,
I hope you will remember
kisses on booboos
and singing of songs.

When you think of me,
I hope you will remember
words of comfort and reassurance,
wiping tears from your eyes,
and bedtime kisses.

When you think of me,
I hope you will remember
giggles and sharing secrets,
snuggles on the couch,
reading books,
and taking walks together.

When you think of me,
I hope you will remember
how my eyes lit up
every time you came home,
and countless "I love you"s.

When you think of me,
I hope you will remember
that I was far from perfect,
but I admitted my mistakes and tried my hardest.

When you think of me,
I hope you will remember
that I'll always cherish
every moment of being your mom.
And that you were, are, and always will be deeply loved.

That love fills me up and forever breathes life into my soul.

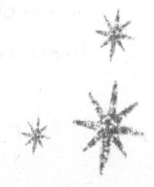

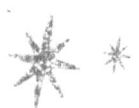

Being the Mother of a Tween or Teen

Being the mother of a tween—nearly a teen—
feels like an endless game of tug-of-war.
I reach towards her,
she yanks away.

She pushes my buttons,
and I know I'm supposed to retreat,
give her space.
But often I engage.

It sometimes feels like
I am losing her.
I extend my hand,
but her grasp is out of reach.

Being the mother of a tween or teen
rips you apart.
It reassembles you,
but the pieces don't quite fit back together.

But even in her darkest hour,
I can still see a flicker—
flashes of what is still there and what's to come.
They dance like shadows behind a curtain.

And those brief glimpses
are like raindrops
to a parched flower.

They give me hope.
They give me strength.

They remind me that she is still my baby.
That she is growing up.
That she needs space to find herself.

But she is still there.
She will always be there.
And I will always be there.

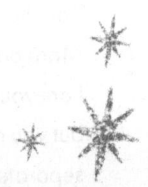

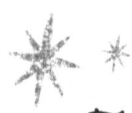

Forever and Always, My Baby You'll Be

Forever and always, my baby you'll be.

I marveled at your little fingers and toes.
Were you really mine?
Your cries pierced my heart like shards of glass.
Exhaustion filled every pore of my body.
I wanted to give you the world,
while grasping the responsibility and privilege
of being your everything.

I never knew I could love this deeply, my baby.

You ran everywhere and got into everything.
Your curiosity was only surpassed by your energy.
I wanted to slow down time,
while speeding up the moments where I felt I was failing you.
You'd look at me, and I would hold back tears of love.
I'd look at you and wonder if I was deserving of you.

I never knew how short the years are, my baby.

There is never a dull moment with you.
Your humor, kindness, and strong will amaze me daily.
More baby teeth have fallen out than I care to admit.
I am your source of comfort and safety,
but you are trying to find your place in this world
separate from me.

I never knew I'd want to relive the past
while yearning for what's to come, my baby.

The years have gone by
quicker than I imagined.
Memories forever etched in my mind.
I am no longer your entire world,
but you will always be mine.

I never knew how hard it would be, my baby.

Except now I know.
I know how bittersweet it is to watch you soar.
I am so proud of the person who stands before me.
I am so honored when you reach your hand out for mine.
I am so grateful that you still let me smother you with kisses.

I never knew I'd want to freeze each time
you ask to be with me, my baby.

You are no longer a baby.
This I know.

But I also know this with the utmost certainty—

Forever and always, my baby you'll be.

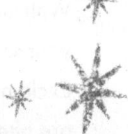

Your Safe Place

When I first held you,
my arms were shelter from every storm
The world was dark and unknown,
and you found solace in my embrace

I was your safe place.

When you were a toddler,
cuts and bruises told the tale
of adventure and mishaps
And when Band-Aids weren't enough
to soothe your pain,
you'd jump into my arms

Because I was your safe place.

As you got older
outer pain was usurped by inner pain
The battles of your heart
could not be eased with kisses
Still, you looked to me
for words of comfort and advice

For I was your safe place.

With that comes the responsibility of being
your source of safety
Exclamations of anger and frustration
are often aimed my way

Cataclysmic behaviors often find their way
into my presence
And although they wound my heart,
I know they are targeting me for a reason

I am your safe place.

Days blur into years:
a kaleidoscope of time
You do not always seek me out,
as growing pains wrap you in isolation
Yet you know I am a breath away
should your words form my name

After all, I am your safe place.

I carry the knowledge
that the sands of time
will wedge their way between us
A detachment in space,
but never in my heart
Because my love for you is your constant

I will always be your safe place.

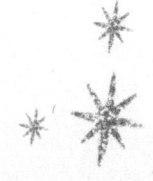

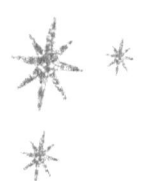

I'm Raising a Child

I'm raising a child who stands up for others
I'm raising a child who asks the kid who is standing alone
to play with her

I'm raising a child who brings money
to give to people who are less fortunate
I'm raising a child who wears her heart on her sleeve

I'm raising a child who volunteers
and writes letters to people that are lonely
I'm raising a child who uses her manners

Good grades are great,
but what matters most to me is that she is a great kid
I'm proud to raise that type of child

No Matter Your Age

No matter your age, I will pray I did right by you.
No matter your age, your well-being will be my priority.
No matter your age, your laughter will warm my heart.
No matter your age, I hope you believe in yourself
as much as I believe in you.

No matter your age, I will worry about you.
No matter your age, I will smile when you're happy
and hurt when you're struggling.
No matter your age, I will offer my shoulder for you to lean on
and my ear to listen.
No matter your age, I will feel gratitude and pride.

No matter your age, I will remind you of your self-worth.
No matter your age, you will always be my baby.
No matter your age, I will be your biggest supporter.
No matter your age, you will always have my heart.

No matter your age, it will be my greatest joy
and my greatest heartbreak to watch you spread your wings.
No matter your age, I will encourage you
to follow your dreams.
No matter your age, I will cherish our time together.
No matter your age, I will love you unconditionally.

No matter your age,
I will always be your mom.
No matter your age.

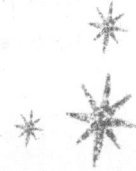

Motherhood Doesn't Get Easier

Motherhood doesn't get easier.

Physical exhaustion turns to mental exhaustion.
Worrying about their scrapes turns
to worrying about their feelings.
Long hours rocking them turn into
long hours waiting for them to return safely.

Motherhood doesn't get easier.

The guilt doesn't fade.
The second guessing doesn't change.
Joy and sorrow continue to waltz
with the firsts and lasts of each milestone.

Motherhood doesn't get easier.
Whether they are babies, toddlers, teenagers, or grown.

Motherhood doesn't get easier.
It just changes.

But the one thing that doesn't change
is how much we love them.

Motherhood doesn't get easier.
Because it is forever.

You Will Always Have My Heart

You are my blessing
My heart and soul
My pride and joy
My greatest gift

My love for you has no restrictions or conditions
My love for you is everlasting and limitless

You will always have my heart
Always.

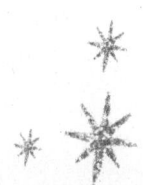

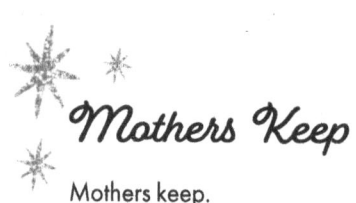

Mothers Keep

Mothers keep.

We keep first curls
We keep baby teeth
We keep photos and videos
We keep countless memories

We keep trophies
We keep art projects
We keep to-do lists
We keep track of schedules

Mothers keep.

We keep trying our best
We keep replaying our mistakes
We keep worrying about our children
We keep showing up

We keep kissing and hugging
We keep praying
We keep wanting to turn back the hands of time
We keep feeling our children's pain

Mothers keep.

We keep cherishing their every smile, every laugh,
every triumph, every embrace
We keep our children in our hearts
We keep loving unconditionally and extraordinarily

And no matter our life circumstances,
or how old our kids may be,
mothers always keep holding on to that love

Because that love is for keeps.

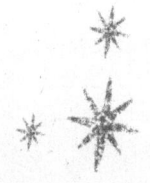

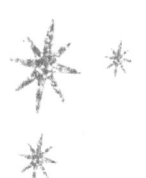

Loving You

I will never claim to have all the answers
I will never be a flawless mom or person

But...
I will always help you through the hard
I will always be your biggest fan and advocate
I will always offer you shelter from life's storms
I will always remind you of your self-worth

I will make countless mistakes
But loving you is the most perfect thing I'll ever do.

I Hope She Knows

I hope she knows how hard I try to be a good mom.
I hope she knows that my anger and frustration
never diminish my love for her.
I hope she knows I don't want her to strive for perfection;
I want her to strive to do her best.
I hope she knows how much joy she brings me
each and every day.

I hope she knows that her laugh lights up my life.
I hope she knows that I will support her no matter her choices,
and no matter where life takes her.
I hope she knows that she is always worthy, just as she is.
I hope she knows that labels, grades, numbers on a scale,
and other people's opinions do not define her.

I hope she knows that the most important relationship
she'll ever have is with herself.
I hope she knows to do what is right and not what is easy.
I hope she knows that it is a privilege to watch her grow,
even though it also breaks my heart.
I hope she knows that she is capable,
and that the sky is the limit for her.

I hope she knows that I feel every pain, tear,
and heartbreak she experiences.
I hope she knows that she is loved beyond measure
and beyond words.

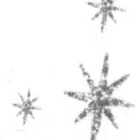

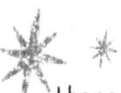

I hope she knows that I will never get it all right,
but I will always keep trying.

I hope she knows.
Even though I tell her.
I hope she knows.

I Never Got to Say Goodbye

I never got to say goodbye.

Every embrace has a release.
Every tomorrow concludes today.

There was no warning that it was over.
There was no foreshadowing of the end.
Only slivers of time that aren't moments
until they're in the rearview mirror.

I long to replay each slideshow of you,
lost but not forgotten.
The pages turned quicker than I imagined.
And although I miss the writing,
I know the words by heart.

Each manifestation of you sparkles brightly.
Each season has its own spectrum of hues,
its own tapestry of light.

A new beginning is born from every ending.
A window opened when doors closed.
The present becomes a distant memory,
for time is truly fleeting.

I never got to say goodbye,
but how could I even if I knew?

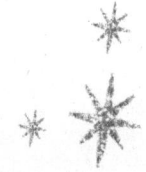

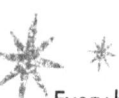

Every beat of my heart—
a reminder of what once was.
Every beat of my heart—
a reminder of the one thing time cannot steal.

I Will Call for You

I will call for you.

When I want you to play with me
When I want you to take care of me
When I can't express my emotions,
but I long for your scent, your voice, your arms

I will call for you.

When I fall and hurt myself
When I am tangled up with my feelings
When I am unable to voice my needs,
I hope you can hear the pleading in my cries

I will call for you.

When I have my first crush
When I have my first love
When I have my first heartbreak
When I feel lost

I will call for you.

When I leave the nest
When I feel uncertain about myself
When I feel uncertain about this world
When I want to feel safe in this world

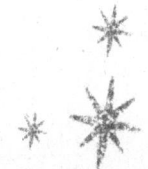

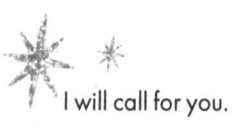

I will call for you.

When I have kids of my own
and the love I feel takes my breath away,
I will understand why you were there

I will understand why you were always there—
when I called for you.

Don't You Know?

I cry because this is the only way I can communicate.
Everything around me seems big and loud,
and I need you in order to feel safe.
I hate when you lay me down
because I find solace in your arms.

I know you're tired, but don't you know?
You are my everything.

I run around, but that is because there is so much to explore.
I am filled with curiosity and ask tons of questions.
I get frustrated because I can't always explain how I'm feeling
and what I'm thinking.
I need you to set limits, while letting me do things myself.

I know you get frustrated, but don't you know?
You are my favorite person in the entire world.

School, hobbies, homework, friends:
My life is filled with other things and people.
I'm figuring out who I am in this world separate from you.
I need you to guide me and support me
as I become more independent.

I know you're not always with me, but don't you know?
You are my anchor and safe place.

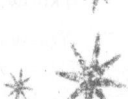

Everything is confusing to me.
My body is changing, and I don't know how to make sense of it.
I don't know if I'm good enough,
and that's hard for me to tell you.
You ask if I'm okay, but I can't find the words
to explain how I'm feeling.

I know I get angry and push you away, but don't you know?
I need you now more than ever.

I don't live at home anymore, but you still check on me.
It sometimes frustrates me, but I know it's only because you care.
Life is busy between working and spending time with friends.
We don't see each other every day,
but you are the one I come to for advice and support.

I know I'm an adult, but don't you know?
I just want to make you proud.

I look at my own child,
and I finally comprehend the depth of your love.
I understand your constant worry and the selflessness required
to let me go.
I just hope I can be as good of a mom as you.

I need your help as I take on the biggest role of my life.

I know I'm a mother now, but don't you know?
You will always be my hero.

Everlasting

When there's gray strands
strewn upon my hair
and I feel fatigue deep within my bones,
when there's a stillness in the air,
my thoughts will constantly drift to you.

I will always recall
the way your laughter
bounced across the walls
and the softness of your skin.
The look of wonder and your mischievous smile
when you found your way
into pots and pans, closets, and items high on shelves.

Your slightly parched lips when you practiced tying your shoes.
Your little hands as you scribbled ferociously.
Your widened eyes as you took in every sound
and every moment.

Memories of raised tempers,
late nights, and mindless routines
will fade into the overwhelming feelings of
love, laughter, and joy.

For the days are long,
but the years,
oh, the years,
they ripped through me
like a tornado.

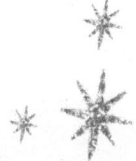

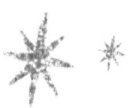

What lives within me,
and I pray within you,
is the knowledge
that you were loved,
and that my love is everlasting.

Final Musings of My Heart

"You shouldn't have a child if you're trying to lower your stress level" is a statement I think we can all agree is accurate. Parenting is wonderful in many ways, but relaxing would never be the adjective I'd use to describe it. In fact, motherhood is the most stressful thing I've ever dealt with in my life (and that's saying something). However, one of the most surprising things I learned about becoming a mother is that motherhood healed me in ways that nothing else could.

When I first became a mother, I was depressed and scared. My husband and I both wanted a baby, and we were overcome with joy when we found out I was pregnant. The fear of miscarriage led my husband to start drinking and taking pills, which continued when our daughter was born. Mix that with a lack of support and absolutely no clue what I was doing, and it was a recipe for disaster. This helpless, innocent baby was counting on me to survive, and the enormity of that made it hard for me to breathe. My own childhood was filled with trauma, so becoming a new parent didn't stir up the happiest of memories. How was I going to be a mother—a good mother—when I was in so much pain myself?

I didn't have the answer then, and frankly, I still don't, but I can share with you what my next move was. I decided to be what I had needed as a child, to give her the unconditional love I never had, and to make sure she never, ever had to question how much she meant to me. I couldn't guarantee much, but loving her was one thing I could do.

And so, I did. I loved her wholeheartedly and without reservation. I poured all the love I had never received into her. I faced all the hardships I'd dealt with as a child and accepted it all for what it was. I couldn't make sure the cycle ended with me unless I faced it head-on.

There were days, hours, and minutes when I felt I would drown from the pressure and exhaustion. The guilt of making wrong choices combined with my lack of confidence as a person and a mother was almost too much to bear. I would crack, but I would never really break, because I found an inner strength and purpose in the eyes of my daughter.

Being the mother of a newborn is hard, until you become the mother of an infant. You can't imagine it being any harder until your child becomes a toddler and is getting into everything. Then you become the mother of a child going to school, and your heartbreak might be the end of you if you didn't adore that child so much. Then that child becomes older and older, and yet, to your amazement, motherhood is still hard: different, but still hard—so hard that the difficulty feels like a storm that ebbs and flows over time. Such storms will change paths and take different shapes, yet you learn how to navigate each one because your love never falters, never wavers, never ceases to exist. And just when you feel like you've gotten a handle on motherhood and the sun is peeking through the clouds, the storm changes course, and you must navigate its ferocity again. Despite these storms, the rainbow that emerges will always take your breath away. It is those shades of emotion when you look into your child's eyes or feel the warmth of their smile that make every obstacle worth it.

I think we all have visions of what motherhood will be like prior to becoming mothers. Our preconceived notions of parenting have a lot to do with our own upbringing. It also can play a role in our choice to become parents and whether we think we'll be good ones.

As I mentioned at the beginning of this book, I am by no means a parenting expert, but one thing I know is that parenting never gets easier. At least, it doesn't for me. The only thing I can count on is being the best I can be during every twist and turn. My best varies all the time because I am human with my own mountains of issues to deal with, but I try. Boy, do I try. And maybe, just maybe, I can break the spell of generations past in the process.

Whether you had a wonderful childhood or not, whether you are a bit of a mess or not, we all are imperfect. There are hard truths we all must face, as motherhood has a way of holding up a mirror to the parts of ourselves that are wounded. We can turn around and ignore them, but the glare of our reflection will always be there.

I am not claiming to be a fully healed person—far from it. What I am is a person who is constantly trying to work on myself. I make mistakes, and then I make some more. Some of them are inevitable; what human doesn't make them? Some are patterns that are simple to fix, and others are years in the making. I will be working on myself until the day I die, but I think half the battle is the willingness to try.

My child has witnessed things that I wish she hadn't. There was chaos and toxicity; there were screams and door slams. Maybe you were raised in a house like that; maybe your house is like that now. We all have regrets and skeletons in our closet. I am airing mine in hopes of showing others that whatever happened in the past or is happening in the present does not have to dictate our future. To quote singer Natasha Bedingfield, "The rest is still unwritten."

If you're reading this book, I'm willing to bet that you love your kid with all your heart, too. I'm also willing to bet (and I'm not a gambler) that you are doing your best to face some of your own inner demons. We are our children's role models, but they are ours as well. We want to be better because of them and for them.

I write because it helps me to express my innermost feelings. For a long time, all I wrote about was pain and sadness. When I had my daughter, a part of me was awakened; a part filled with hope, a part filled with meaning. A part filled with insurmountable love.

Time changes, and my daughter is now heading into teendom. I have no idea what this next phase of life will bring. I do know that it will have its own unique set of challenges and that I will have to learn as I go.

What I also know is that I now write because there is someone besides myself to worry about and to protect. And when I doubt myself and my inner demons rear their ugly heads, I will read these poems and remind myself that something beautiful came out of my life (see image below). I hope you will do so, too.

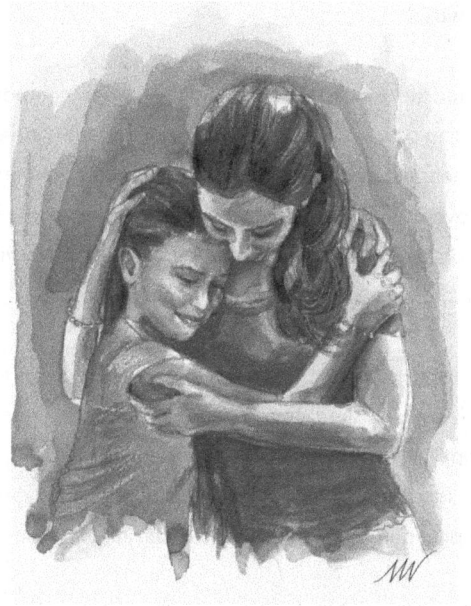

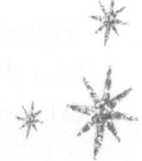

Final Musings of My Heart

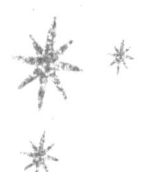

Conclusion

"Why do you keep doing this?" my daughter asked me as I frowned. I had read yet another rejection letter, and the disappointment was coming off me in waves. I looked at her, and there was so much I wanted to say. I chose to keep it brief. "Because this is my dream, and dreams should not be thrown away."

I've learned that writing a book is not the hardest component of the writing process. Getting the book published is indeed the most challenging and discouraging part. Once it dawned on me that my love of writing poetry could be channeled into a book, I dreamt of the day that I could hold it in my hands. My vision, however, didn't mean it was other people's vision.

Poetry is not an easy genre to get published. In fact, it is the hardest. Most publishers won't even bother to read your manuscript if it is poetry. It was hard enough to be taken seriously as a first-time author, but I was also trying to get a manuscript of autobiographical poetry out into the world.

This book is years in the making. Just as being a mother is a labor of love, so was this book. I've watched my daughter grow as I wove these poems together. I faced self-doubt, worry, frustration, and moments of questioning my worth as a writer as well as a mother.

I hope my child always follows her heart and her dreams. They are worth following. Your dreams, dear reader, are worth following, too. The truth is that dreams aren't for the faint of heart. Like parenting, the most wonderful things in life are often the hardest.

I am so grateful to you for being a part of my dream becoming a reality. Your purchase of this book means the world to me. The world of publishing is not an easy one to break into, and it truly helps if you leave a positive review on Amazon and spread the word about my book. Thank you!

Although this book is coming to an end, my hope is that this is just the beginning for me as a published author. I have visions of future books, and I'd love to know what kinds of poems you would like to see from me. Please email me at survivingmomblog@gmail.com to let me know! I read and respond to all my emails, and I'd be thrilled to hear from you.

I'm on social media as well, so don't forget to follow me at Facebook.com/survivmomblog, Instagram.com/survivingmomblog, and tiktok.com/@randilatzman. I also have a free monthly newsletter, so you can join me over there at survivingmomblog.com/subscribe.

Thank you for holding my heart in your hands as you've read this book. I hope my words have brought comfort and reassurance to your heart as well.

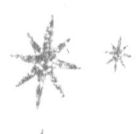

Acknowledgments from This Mother's Heart

How do I begin to show my appreciation for so many who helped shape me and this book?

To Brenda and the entire Mango team, thank you for all your hard work and for putting my book out into the world. Thank you for believing in me and my web of feelings that I call poems. Poetry is a genre that most publishers hide from, but you ran towards me instead of away. I will always be grateful.

To the lovely and talented Becca Anderson. I am so honored to have your words open the door for mine. Thank you for your support and wisdom. Thank you for using your voice to champion for others.

To Leslie and the Her View from Home writers, I remember being awed by this group of writers and instantly feeling like an imposter. However, you all welcomed me and made me feel like I belonged. You made me feel like my writing belonged. I am grateful for the many friendships I've forged though this incredible community. Thank you for all your support, advice, and encouragement.

To Dani, my mentor, you took me under your wing when I didn't know anything about Facebook and could barely put a post online. Thank you for your advice, tips, support, and connections. I am so grateful for the friendship that blossomed from a message, and I'm honored to have you in my corner.

To Melissa, my oldest and dearest friend of over thirty years: Many of my favorite memories have you in them. From taking walks around the neighborhood, to liking the same boy as CITs, to crazy discoveries in the restroom of a club, we've been through a lot together. I'm still honored that David called me to help pick your outfit the day of your proposal, and does "schmutz" gross you out if I type it instead of saying it? Despite the distance, hectic schedules, and life circumstances, we've always found a way to stay connected. I guess you should now get the nickname "Professor." I love you, and I'm so proud of all your accomplishments.

To my in-laws, thank you for being so supportive and encouraging about this crazy gig I call writing. The enthusiasm and support you gave me when I told you about this book is something I will always treasure. I love you both and am grateful to call you my other parents.

To my father, thank you for taking the flight to Atlanta every month so I can hug you and vent about my latest shenanigans in person. Your wit, love for animals, intelligence,

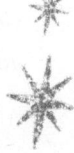

and ability to listen to the TV on the lowest volume possible never cease to amaze me. I love you, Daddy.

To my sister, Kari, and to my siblings-in-law Lauren, Joe, Eric, and Jacky, you all have a special place in my heart. Each of you have brightened my life by being a part of it. Kari, I still think of you as a little girl with a polka-dot dress and handbag, but I am so proud of the wife and mother you've become. The best part of my childhood was having you as my sister. I love you always.

To my mom, it would be impossible to write a book about motherhood without acknowledging you. I know you did the best you could. You are with me every time I sing Brielle one of the many songs you taught me and when I attempt to teach her "The Spades Go" hand game. I remember you rubbing my back and tummy when I was sick. I remember you whispering to me while we cuddled in your bed. I remember the ski trip we took (how did those little kids get on that lift, and why couldn't I get back up when I fell?), and I remember when the two of us went by ourselves to Kutchers. You played a huge role in shaping the person and mother I am today. There is so much I admire about you, and I love you.

To my readers, I am beyond humbled that you purchased my book. Your feedback and words of encouragement warm my heart and breathe life into this overly exhausted soul. It was your inquiries about a book that gave me the final push to enter the world of publishing. I am forever grateful for allowing me into your homes and your heart. From the bottom of mine, thank you.

To my husband, Matt, there are no words to express my love and gratitude. You were instrumental in this book becoming a reality. From creating the website that started it all to helping me navigate social media, designing my webpage when I wanted it to be more of an author's page, answering my endless questions about formatting, and being a beta reader for me, you have been a jack of endless trades (whether you've liked it or not). You believed in me when I didn't believe in myself. You encouraged me to write more pages when I didn't think I had any words left in me. The day I became your wife will always be the best day of my life. My home is wherever you are. I love you forever.

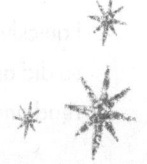

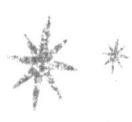

About the Author

One of the most frequent stories I've heard about me was one that happened when I was twenty-one months old. My mother took me to a speech pathologist because I wasn't talking much. The speech pathologist evaluated me, and she called my mother to discuss her concern about my delay. In true Randi fashion, I started talking a few months later and have never stopped talking since (although I'm inherently shy).

When I was three, I made my father promise me he would never die. I was strong-willed and determined (I guess the joke's on me now that my daughter possesses those traits), and my dad conceded. Still a strong-willed and determined adult, I often remind him of his promise.

I was a perfectionist and competitive from an early age. My first-grade teacher announced a reading contest. The child who read the most books would get a box of crayons. I was determined to win. I loved reading, *and* I could get a box of crayons? It was a win-win.

I quickly gathered tallies next to my name. The problem was, so did another girl named "Kelly." For every book I read, Kelly read one. Kelly and I read two books a day for the next few weeks, while the other kids eventually tapered off. Even at six, these kids knew when it was time to throw in the towel. The teacher eventually realized that this was getting out of hand, and she called off the contest. The way the two of us were behaving, you would think the prize was a trip to Disneyland.

Although I lost out on the box of crayons, I did not lose my love of reading and writing. I got swept away by the words and images in my mind. I was such an avid reader that one of my punishments was having my books taken away (yes, you read that correctly). I found that writing was therapeutic for me, and I turned to poetry to articulate my innermost feelings.

When I was eleven, I was accepted into a middle school based on my talent for creative writing. I was exposed to a variety of genres, but poetry always had a special place in my heart. I continued to write poems to help me get through the pain I felt throughout my childhood, and I still have many of them somewhere in my house to this day.

I always wore my heart on my sleeve, crying at any and all shows (nobody liked going to the movies with me) and even at many a commercial. I was sensitive and felt very deeply. I guess some things never change.

I never thought a career in writing was attainable, so I decided to be a lawyer. *Matlock* (remember him?) was one of my favorite shows, and I wanted to be just like him. I have a strong moral compass and wanted to help those who couldn't help themselves. I had notions of saving the world, not realizing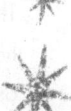

that a defense lawyer must also defend guilty people. Once that notion dawned on me, I was back to the drawing board.

I majored in Speech Language Pathology and Audiology in college (it is a coincidence that I was evaluated by one as a child) and earned my masters in Speech Pathology. I provided services to children in various preschool settings. I always loved children, and I worked with them in some capacity from the time I was a teenager.

When I had my daughter, I stopped working to be a stay-at-home mom. She became my only (and favorite) client, and I focused on being the best mother I could be to her.

When COVID hit, I felt insurmountable helplessness about the lack of support many were experiencing during the pandemic. I wanted to bring comfort to others, but how? I started writing publicly to provide connections for others during a time when there was none. Eventually that turned into starting a Facebook page, which naturally evolved into combining my love for my daughter with my first love, poetry.

If you told me that writing would become my career, I would have simultaneously laughed and shaken my head. The notion never crossed my mind, especially as I was entering my fifth decade of life.

This decade has been one of many changes. White strands have turned up in my hair (wasn't it supposed to turn gray first?), as well as fine (ish?) lines around my eyes and mouth and a toe that aches when it's cold outside. Doctors now blame most of my ailments on "age." Perimenopause is the biggest thing to pop up on my social media feed (was that term around when I was growing up?). My new BFFs are face creams.

I think the biggest changes have taken place internally. I've gained awareness that my time on this planet is finite. Just like the container of strawberries in my fridge, I have an expiration date.

This internal shift is partly due to being sandwiched between two generations that are each getting older and depending on me. For a long time, it was just my child that required my care. Now that my daughter is older, I must adjust to being the mom of a hormonal tween (two words I'll never get used to writing or saying). However, my child isn't the only one who is getting older. Over the last few years, there has been an increased concern for my parents. (My in-laws count as my parents, too.)

After years of being a stay-at-home mom, I never fathomed starting such an exciting and new chapter of my life. I must remind myself that it wasn't twenty-ish Randi or thirty-ish Randi that signed a book deal. It was this forty-year-old who can't-sit-for-too-long-because-it-hurts-my-back who made those dreams a reality. Life sometimes throws us a bouquet of flowers when we least expect it, and I am so grateful I caught it.

I currently reside in Atlanta, Georgia with my daughter and husband, a dog, and two cats. If I'm not taking care of my daughter, watching too much reality TV with my husband, or cleaning, you'll find me attempting to navigate the computer where I continue to write. The why to the last part is on the next page.

I Was the Girl That Wrote

I was the girl that wrote.

I wrote to express the pain I felt.
I wrote to feel less alone in this world.
I wrote because it gave me a voice.
I wrote because I was trying to process
a world filled with confusion.

I was the girl that wrote.

I wrote to put a harmony to a song without any rhythm.
I wrote to find solace within my words.
I wrote to channel the echoes of the walls within me.
I wrote because I longed to be heard.

I was the girl that wrote.

When there was loneliness in my heart.
When there was emptiness in my soul.
When there were questions that didn't have answers.

I was the girl that wrote.

So that I could hold onto hope.
So that I could see light at the end of the tunnel.
So that I could see the beauty amidst the cacophony of pain.

I am the girl that writes
so that the broken pieces within me can have purpose.

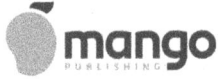

Mango Publishing, established in 2014, publishes an eclectic list of books by diverse authors—both new and established voices—on topics ranging from business, personal growth, women's empowerment, LGBTQ studies, health, and spirituality to history, popular culture, time management, decluttering, lifestyle, mental wellness, aging, and sustainable living. We were named 2019 and 2020's #1 fastest growing independent publisher by *Publishers Weekly*. Our success is driven by our main goal, which is to publish high-quality books that will entertain readers as well as make a positive difference in their lives.

Our readers are our most important resource; we value your input, suggestions, and ideas. We'd love to hear from you—after all, we are publishing books for you!

Please stay in touch with us and follow us at:

Facebook: Mango Publishing
Twitter: @MangoPublishing
Instagram: @MangoPublishing
LinkedIn: Mango Publishing
Pinterest: Mango Publishing
Newsletter: mangopublishinggroup.com/newsletter

Join us on Mango's journey to reinvent publishing, one book at a time.